HANDBOOK of
Radiographic
Positioning
AND Techniques

John P. Lampignano, MEd, R.T. (R)(CT)(ARRT)
Leslie E. Kendrick, MS, R.T. (R)(CT)(MR)(ARRT)

ELSEVIER

Elsevier
3251 Riverport Lane
St. Louis, Missouri 63043

HANDBOOK OF RADIOGRAPHIC POSITIONING
AND TECHNIQUES, ELEVENTH EDITION   ISBN: 978-0-323-93616-3

Notice

Practitioners and researchers must always rely on their own experience and knowledge in evaluating and using any information, methods, compounds or experiments described herein. Because of rapid advances in the medical sciences, in particular, independent verification of diagnoses and drug dosages should be made. To the fullest extent of the law, no responsibility is assumed by Elsevier, authors, editors or contributors for any injury and/or damage to persons or property as a matter of products liability, negligence or otherwise, or from any use or operation of any methods, products, instructions, or ideas contained in the material herein.

Previous editions copyrighted 2021, 2018 by Elsevier, Inc.
Previous edition copyrighted 2014 by Mosby, an imprint of Elsevier Inc.
Previous edition copyrighted 2010 by Mosby, Inc., an affiliate of Elsevier Inc.
Previous editions copyrighted 2002, 1999, 1995, 1994 by Kenneth L. Bontrager

Content Strategist: Meg Benson
Sr. Content Development Specialist: Tina Kaemmerer
Publishing Services Manager: Deepthi Unni
Project Manager: Sindhuraj Thulasingam
Cover Design: Amy Buxton

Printed in India

Last digit is the print number:
9 8 7 6 5 4 3 2 1

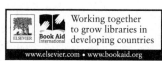

Working together
to grow libraries in
developing countries

www.elsevier.com • www.bookaid.org

Preface

This pocket handbook was first developed by Kenneth Bontrager in 1994 as a response to the need felt by students and technologists for a more thorough but still practical pocket guide covering the applied aspects of radiographic positioning and techniques (exposure factors). Today, this compact and durable pocket-sized handbook includes a review of all the common imaging procedures, yet it is small enough to be easily carried in clinical situations. Space is included for writing personal notes and exposure factors that technologists find are optimal for specific equipment or in certain rooms or departments. Careful attention has been given to ensure the information on positioning in the textbook is reflected accurately in the handbook.

Positioning descriptions and photographs are provided for each projection/position, along with CR locations, degrees of obliquity, specific CR angles, AEC cell locations, and suggested kVp ranges. A quick review of this information before beginning a procedure can ensure the examination is being correctly performed, reducing the need for repeat exposures as a result of poor positioning or improper exposure factors.

Standard Radiographic Image and Evaluation Criteria
The eleventh edition of this handbook includes a standard, well-positioned radiograph with each position described. Also added is a brief summary of quality factors to use an image evaluation matrix. Viewing this radiograph and comparing it with the list of evaluation criteria leads users through a critique of the image they are viewing for comparison to this standard.

Acknowledgments

Meg Benson, Tina Kaemmerer, and Sindhuraj Thulasingam with Elsevier Publishing were instrumental in providing support, guidance, and the resources in the redesign and publishing of the pocket handbook. We are most indebted to our current and former students, fellow technologists, and those many educators throughout the United States and in the international imaging community who challenged and inspired us. We thank you and hope this pocket handbook continues to be a valuable resource in improving and maintaining the high level radiographic imaging for which we all strive.

John and Leslie

Contents

Contents

Explanations for Use

This handbook is intended to be a quick reference and review of radiographic positioning and procedures. It is not intended to replace the positioning techniques described in the Radiographic Positioning and Related Anatomy textbook. Rather, it is an ancillary tool that provides the technologist a quick review of the critical elements on positioning, central ray (CR), location, kilovoltage peak (kVp) ranges, and methods for reducing patient dose. These critical elements include:

Radiation protection: Certain radiation protection practices and shielding descriptions are included with each projection, and it is the responsibility of the technologist to ensure that shielding of radiosensitive tissues, collimation, and proper exposure factors are applied for each examination as per policy and local regulations. Department policies may state whether gonadal shielding should be used. Recommendations **for reducing patient dose are described in Appendix A**.

kVp ranges: Suggested kVp ranges are stated for each projection. These are recommendations based on best practices and validated by imaging experts. **These kVp ranges may not apply to every department protocol or imaging systems employed**. The technologist should consult with their radiation safety officer or supervisor to determine appropriate kVp ranges for their clinical setting.

Chapter title pages: The list of projections with page numbers is at the beginning of each chapter for ease in locating specific projections and as a reference for marking the basic department routines for each examination. A small check (✓) can be placed in the box by each projection that is part of the preferred departmental routine. Each projection is also followed by either an (**R**) or a (**S**) for a suggested departmental **routine** or **special**.

Standard Radiographic Image and Evaluation Criteria: Associated with each positioning page is a radiograph of the projection. These radiographs demonstrate the critical anatomy that must be visualized. A list of **evaluation criteria** is provided for the technologists to critique the images they have produced.

Each positioning page has a format similar to this sample page.

1. Recommended automatic exposure control (AEC) chamber(s) (darkened R and L upper cells indicated on this PA chest example). **Note:** Verify AEC chamber selection with department before employing.

2. Recommended collimation field size with CR location in center.

3. IR alignment recommended for an average adult, placed portrait or landscape in reference to the anatomy of interest. Grid or nongrid.

4. Patient position description.

5. CR location and CR angle.

6. Suggested source to image receptor distance (SID) range.

7. Recommendations for patient respiration during image exposure.

8. Suggested kVp ranges. (Pencil in kVp range for your imaging systems.)

9. Exposure and imaging factors to be filled in (in pencil) as determined best for small (S), medium (M), or large (L) patients.

10. Corresponding page number in the textbook for detailed information on the projection.

PA: Chest

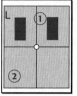
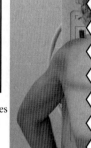

- 14 × 17 inches (35 × 43 cm)
3. portrait or landscape
- Grid

Fig. 1.3 PA chest (vertebra prominens)

Position (4)
- Erect, chin raised, hands on hips, rotated forward against IR
- Center CR to the center of the lu patients with accurate collimation
- Center thorax bilaterally to IR b both sides; ensure there is **no rot** midcoronal plane parallel to the

Central Ray: CR ⊥ to IR, centered (5) 20 cm) below vertebra prominen

SID: 72 inches (180 cm) (6)

Collimation field size: Collimate on (top border of illuminated field shou prominens, and lateral border shoul

Respiration: (7) Expose at end of **se**

kVp Range: (8)

(9)	cm	kVp	mA	Time
S				
M				
L				

(10) Textbook, 11th

Chapter 1

Chest

(R) Routine, (S) Special

Positioning Considerations and Radiation Protection
Collimation

Careful collimation is important in chest radiography. Restricting the primary x-ray beam by collimation not only reduces patient dose by reducing the volume of tissue irradiated but also improves image quality by reducing scatter radiation.

Correct CR Location

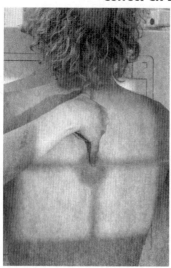

Fig. 1.1 Correct CR location for PA projection.

Correct CR location to the midchest (T7) allows for accurate collimation and protection of the upper radiosensitive region of the neck area. It also prevents exposure to the dense abdominal area below the diaphragm, which produces scatter and secondary radiation to the radiosensitive reproductive organs.

T7 for the **PA chest** can be located posteriorly in reference to C7, the **vertebra prominens**. Level of T7 is 7–8 inches (18–20 cm) below the vertebra prominens. Fig. 1.2).

The CR for the **AP chest** is 3–4 inches (8–11 cm) below the **jugular notch** and angled 3°–5° caudad (CR perpendicular to midsternum). (Fig. 1.3)

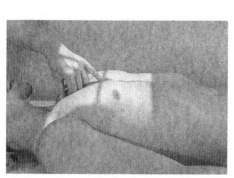

Fig. 1.2 Correct CR location for AP projection.

Radiation Protection

- Exposure factor selection should be optimized in accordance with ALARA.
- Collimate on four sides to anatomy of interest when feasible.
- Radiologic technologists should follow local regulations, department policy and protocol in the use of shielding.

Digital Imaging Considerations

The following technical factors will reduce dose to the patient and improve image quality.

Collimation Field Size

Close collimation reduces dose to the patient and scatter radiation reaching the image receptor.

Accurate Centering

Because of the exposure factors used for the digital image receptor, it is important that the body part and central ray (CR) be accurately centered to the IR. In chest imaging, this involves centering the CR to the center of the lung fields.

Exposure Factors

Digital systems are known for wide exposure latitude, utilizing a broad range of exposure factors (kVp and mAs). However, the ALARA principle must still be followed; therefore, the highest kVp and lowest mAs, consistent with optimal image quality, should be used.

Exposure

The technologist must check the exposure indicator to verify that the exposure factors used were in the correct range to ensure optimal image receptor exposure and contrast with the least radiation to the patient.

Grids

As a general rule, in chest radiography, the use of high kVp (>100) **requires the use of a grid**. Virtual grid technology may eliminate the need for a physical grid.

Textbook, 11th ed, p. 41

PA: Chest

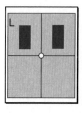

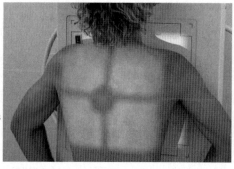

- 14 × 17 inches (35 × 43 cm) portrait or landscape
- Grid

Fig. 1.3 PA chest (CR ~8 inches [20 cm] below vertebra prominens) (average female, 7 inches [18 cm]).

Position

- Erect, chin raised, hands on hips with palms out, shoulders rotated forward against IR
- Center CR to the center of the lung fields on **all types** of patients with accurate collimation on both top and bottom.
- Center thorax bilaterally to IR borders with equal margins on both sides; ensure there is **no rotation** of thorax by placing the midcoronal plane parallel to the IR.

Central Ray: CR ⊥ to IR, centered to T7, or 7–8 inches (18–20 cm) below vertebra prominens (or inferior angle of scapula)

SID: 72 inches (180 cm)

Collimation field size: Collimate on four sides to area of lung fields (top border of illuminated field should be to the level of vertebra prominens, and lateral border should be to outer skin margins).

Respiration: Expose at end of **second full inspiration**.

	cm	kVp	mA	Time	mAs	SID	Exposure Indicator
S							
M							
L							

kVp Range: 110–125

Textbook, 11th ed, p. 88

Lateral: Chest

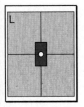

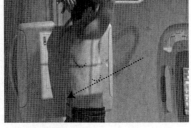

Fig. 1.4 Left lateral chest.

- 14 × 17 inches (35 × 43 cm) portrait
- Grid

Position
- Erect, **left side** against IR (unless right lateral is indicated)
- Arms raised above head, chin up
- **True lateral**, no rotation or tilt; midsagittal plane parallel to IR (do not push hips in against the IR holder)
- Thorax centered to CR, and to IR anteriorly and posteriorly

Central Ray: CR ⊥ to IR, centered to midthorax at level of T7; generally, IR and CR should be lowered ≈1 inches (2.5 cm) from PA on average patient.

SID: 72 inches (180 cm)

Collimation field size: Collimate on four sides to area of lung fields (top border of light field to level of vertebra prominens).

Respiration: Expose at end of **second full inspiration**.

	cm	kVp	mA	Time	mAs	SID	Exposure Indicator
kVp Range:						110–125	
S							
M							
L							

Textbook, 11th ed, p. 90

Lateral (Wheelchair or Stretcher): Chest

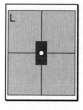

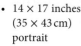

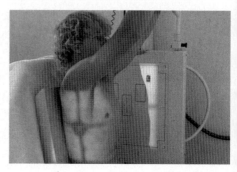

- 14 × 17 inches
  (35 × 43 cm)
  portrait
- Grid

Fig. 1.5 Left lateral on stretcher.

Position

- Erect, on stretcher or in wheelchair
- Arms crossed above head, or hold on to arm support
- Center thorax to CR, and to IR anteriorly and posteriorly.
- No rotation or tilt, midsagittal plane parallel to IR, chin extended upward

Central Ray

- CR ⊥ to IR, centered to midthorax at level of T7 (3 to 4 inches [8 to 10 cm] below level of jugular notch)

SID: 72 inches (180 cm)

Collimation field size: Collimate on four sides to area of lung fields (top border of light field to level of vertebra prominens).

Respiration: Expose at end of **second full inspiration**.

kVp Range:					110–125	
	cm	kVp	mA	Time	mAs	SID	Exposure Indicator
S							
M							
L							

Textbook, 11th ed, p. 91

PA (AP): Chest

Evaluation Criteria
Anatomy Demonstrated
- Both lungs from apices to costophrenic angles, and both lateral borders of ribs
- Ten ribs demonstrated above the diaphragm

Position
- Chin sufficiently elevated and forward shoulder rotation to prevent superimposition of scapulae over lung fields

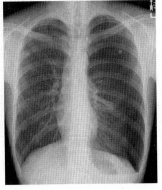

Fig. 1.6 PA chest.

Chest

- No rotation, SC joints and lateral rib margins equal distance from midline of spine

Exposure
- No motion, sharp outlines of rib margins, diaphragm, heart borders, and sharp lung markings
- Optimal image receptor exposure and contrast to visualize fine vascular markings within lungs, faint outlines of midthoracic and upper thoracic vertebrae and posterior ribs visible through heart and mediastinal structures

Lateral: Chest

Evaluation Criteria

Anatomy Demonstrated

- Entire lungs from apices to costophrenic angles, from sternum to posterior ribs

Position

- Chin and arms elevated to prevent superimposing apices
- No rotation, posterior ribs and costophrenic angle on side away from IR projected slightly (¼ to ½ inch

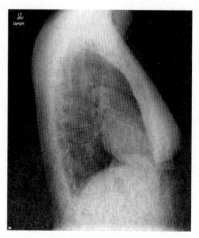

Fig. 1.7 Lateral chest.

[or about 1 cm] posterior because of divergent rays)
- The hilar region should be in the approximate center of the IR.

Exposure

- No motion, sharp outlines of diaphragm and lung markings
- Sufficient exposure of long-scale contrast to visualize rib outlines and lung markings through heart shadow **and upper lung areas** without overexposing other regions of the lungs

Lateral Decubitus: Chest

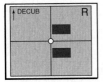

- 14 × 17 inches (35 × 43 cm) landscape with respect to patient position
- Grid

Fig. 1.8 Left lateral decubitus chest (AP).

Position
- Patient on side (R or L, see *Note*) with radiolucent pad under patient
- Ensure that stretcher does not move (lock wheels).
- Chin extended and both arms raised above head to clear lung field; back of patient firmly against IR
- True AP, no rotation, patient centered to CR at level of T7 CR (top of IR is approximately 1 inch [2.5 cm] above vertebra prominens)

Central Ray: CR horizontal to T7, 3–4 inches (8–10 cm) below jugular notch

SID: 72 inches (180 cm) with wall bucky; 40–44 inches (100–110 cm) with erect table and bucky

Collimation field size: Collimate on four sides to area of lung fields (top border of light field to level of vertebra prominens).

Respiration: End of **second full inspiration**

Note: For possible fluid (pleural effusion), suspected side down; possible air (pneumothorax), suspected side up

	cm	kVp	mA	Time	mAs	SID	Exposure Indicator
kVp Range:				**110–125**			
S							
M							
L							

Textbook, 11th ed, p. 93

AP Lordotic: Chest

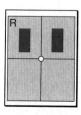

- 14 × 17 inches (35 × 43 cm) portrait or landscape
- Grid

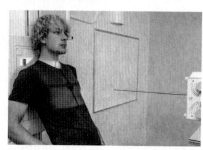

Fig. 1.9 AP lordotic (best demonstrates apices of lungs).

Position

- Patient stands ≈1 ft (30 cm) away from IR, leans back with shoulders, neck, and back of head against IR.
- Hands on hips, palms out, shoulders rolled forward

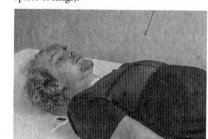

Fig. 1.10 AP axial supine, CR 15–20° cephalad.

- Center midsagittal plane to CR; top of **IR** should be 3 inches (7–8 cm) above shoulders.

Central Ray: CR ⊥ to IR, centered to midsternum (3–4 inches [9 cm] below jugular notch)

SID: 72 inches (180 cm)

Collimation field size: Collimate on four sides to area of lung fields (top border of light field to level of vertebra prominens).

Respiration: End of **second full inspiration**

Note: If patient is too weak and unstable or is unable to assume the erect lordotic position, perform AP semiaxial projection with 15°–20° cephalad angle.

kVp Range:					110–125		
	cm	kVp	mA	Time	mAs	SID	Exposure Indicator
S							
M							
L							

Lateral Decubitus: Chest

Evaluation Criteria
Anatomy
Demonstrated
- Entire lung fields, including apices both costophrenic angles and lateral borders of ribs

Position: No rotation, equal distance from vertebral column to the lateral borders of the ribs on both sides; SC joints should be the

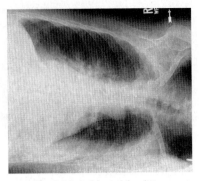

Fig. 1.11 Left lateral decubitus.

same distance from the vertebral column. Arms should not superimpose upper lungs. Collimation field (CR) should be centered to the area of T7 on average-sized patients.

Exposure
- **No motion**; diaphragm, ribs, heart borders, and lung markings appear sharp.
- Optimal image receptor exposure and contrast should result in faint visualization of vertebrae and ribs through heart shadow.

AP Lordotic: Chest

Evaluation Criteria

Anatomy Demonstrated

- Entire lung fields; include clavicles, which should appear above apices

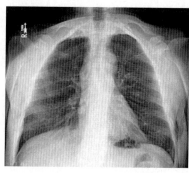

Fig. 1.12 AP lordotic chest.

Position

- Clavicles appear nearly horizontal, superior to apices.
- Ribs appear distorted, with posterior ribs appearing nearly horizontal and superimposing anterior ribs.
- No rotation as evident by equal distance between medial ends of clavicles and lateral borders of ribs and midline of spine

Exposure

- No motion; diaphragm, heart, and rib outlines appear sharp.
- Optimal image receptor exposure and contrast to visualize faint vascular markings of lungs, especially in region of the apices and upper lungs

Anterior Oblique (RAO and LAO): Chest

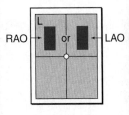

RAO ← | or | → LAO

- 14 × 17 inches (35 × 43 cm) portrait
- Grid

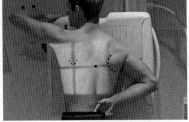

Fig. 1.13 45° RAO.

Position
- Erect, rotated 45°, right anterior shoulder against IR for RAO and rotated 45° with left anterior shoulder against IR for LAO (Certain heart studies require LAO, 60° rotation from PA.)
- Alternative posterior oblique positions can be performed. LPO is best demonstrated left thorax and RPO the right thorax.
- Arm away from IR up resting on head or on IR holder
- Arm nearest IR down on hip, patient looking straight ahead and chin raised
- Center thorax laterally to IR margins; vertically to CR at T7.

Central Ray: CR ⊥ to IR, centered to level of T7 (7–8 inches [8–10 cm] below level of vertebra prominens) midway between midsagittal plane and lateral margin of thorax

SID: 72 inches (180 cm)

Collimation field size: Collimate on four sides to area of lung fields (top border of light field to level of vertebra prominens).

Respiration: End of **second full inspiration**

	cm	kVp	mA	Time	mAs	SID	Exposure Indicator
S							
M							
L							

kVp Range: 110–125

Textbook, 11th ed, p. 95

Evaluation Criteria
Anatomy Demonstrated
- Included both lung fields from apices to costophrenic angles; RAO will elongate left thorax, and LAO will elongate right thorax.

Position
- With 45° rotation, distance from outer rib margins to vertebral column on side farthest from IR should be approximately two times distance of side closest to IR.

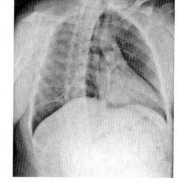

Fig. 1.14 45° RAO.

Exposure
- No motion; diaphragm and rib margins appear sharp.
- Vascular markings throughout lungs and rib outlines visualized faintly through heart
- Optimal image receptor exposure and contrast to allow visualization of vascular markings throughout the lungs and rib outlines except

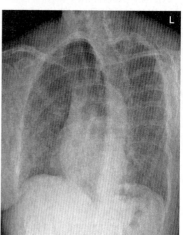

Fig. 1.15 45° LAO.

through the densest regions of the heart.

Notes
- Anterior oblique positions best demonstrate the side farthest from IR. Posterior oblique positions best demonstrate the side closest to IR.
- Less rotation (15°–20°) may allow better visualization of areas of lungs for possible pulmonary disease.

AP and Lateral: Upper Airway
Trachea and Larynx

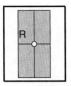

- 10 × 12 inches (24 × 30 cm) portrait
- Grid

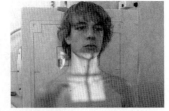

Fig. 1.16 AP upper airway.

Position

- Erect, seated, or standing, center upper airway to CR
- Arms down; elevate mandible to level of base of the skull
- Arms down, chin raised slightly
- Lateral: depress shoulders, and pull shoulders back

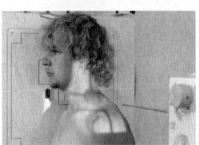

Fig. 1.17 Lateral upper airway.

- Position patient to center upper airway to CR and to center of IR (larynx and trachea lie anterior to cervical and thoracic vertebrae).

Central Ray: CR ⊥ to IR, centered to level of C6 or C7, midway between the laryngeal prominence of the thyroid cartilage and the jugular notch

SID: 72 inches (180 cm)

Collimation field size: Collimate to region of soft tissue neck.

Respiration: Expose during slow, deep inspiration.

	cm	kVp	mA	Time	mAs	SID	Exposure Indicator
kVp Range:					75–85		
S							
M							
L							

Textbook, 11th ed, pp. 98 and 99

AP and Lateral: Upper Airway

Evaluation Criteria

Anatomy Demonstrated:

AP and Lateral

- Soft tissue neck anatomy to include larynx and trachea, filled with air

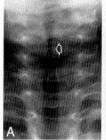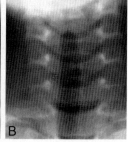

Fig. 1.18 AP upper airway (A. Closed glottis B. Open glottis).

Position:

AP

- No rotation, symmetric appearance of SC joints
- Mandible superimposes base of skull.

Lateral

- To visualize neck region, include external auditory meatus at upper border of image.
- If distal larynx and trachea is of primary interest, the IR and CR should be lowered to place the CR at the upper jugular notch (T1-2).

Exposure:

AP and Lateral

- Optimal image receptor exposure and contrast includes a soft tissue technique wherein the air-filled larynx and upper trachea are not overexposed.
- Cervical vertebrae appear underexposed.

Fig. 1.19 Lateral upper airway.

AP (Tabletop): Pediatric Chest

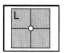

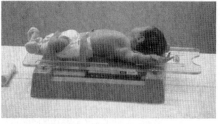

- 8 × 10 inches or 10 × 12 inches (18 × 24 cm or 24 × 30 cm) landscape

Fig. 1.20 Immobilization device.

- Nongrid; grid with digital systems when it cannot be removed

Position
- Supine, arms and legs extended, tape and sandbags or other immobilization of arms and legs
- No rotation of thorax, shield gonadal region as specified by department policy
- IR and thorax centered to CR, with shoulders 2 inches (5 cm) below top of IR

Central Ray: CR ⊥ to IR, centered to the midsagittal plane at the **level of midthorax**, mammillary (nipple) line

SID: Minimum 50–60 inches (125–150 cm); x-ray tube raised as high as possible

Collimation field size: Closely collimate on four sides to outer chest margins.

Respiration: Second full inspiration; if crying, time the exposure at full inhalation.

Note: If parental assistance is necessary, have parent hold child's arms overhead tilting head back with one hand and holding down legs with other hand (provide lead apron and gloves).

	cm	kVp	mA	Time	mAs	SID	Exposure Indicator
kVp Range:					70–85		
S							
M							
L							

Textbook, 11th ed, p. 639

Erect PA (With Pigg-O-Stat): Pediatric Chest

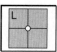

- 8 × 10 inches (18 × 24 cm) or 10 × 12 inches (24 × 30 cm) portrait
- Nongrid or grid with systems when it cannot be removed

Position

- Patient on seat, legs through openings
- Adjust height of seat to place

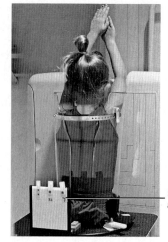

Markers and shield

Fig. 1.21 PA chest (Pigg-O-Stat, for 5-year-old) (DR).

shoulders ~ 1 inch (2.5 cm) below upper margin of IR.
- Raise arms, and gently but firmly place side body clamps to hold raised arms and head in place.
- Set upper border of lead shield with R and L markers 1–2 inches (2.5–5 cm) above level of iliac crest.

Central Ray: CR ⊥ to IR, centered to midlung fields, mammillary (nipple) line

SID: Minimum of 72 inches (180 cm)

Collimation field size: Collimate closely on four sides to outer chest margins.

Respiration: Full inspiration; if crying, expose at full inhalation.

	cm	kVp	mA	Time	mAs	SID	Exposure Indicator
kVp Range:				70–85			
S							
M							
L							

Textbook, 11th ed, p. 640

Chest

Lateral (Tabletop): Pediatric Chest

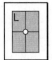

- 8 × 10 inches (18 × 24 cm) or 10 × 12 inches 24 × 30 cm) portrait
- Nongrid or grid with systems when it cannot be removed

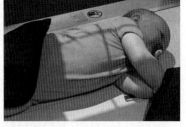

Fig. 1.22 Lateral chest (with tape and sandbags).

Position

- Lying on side (typically left lateral), arms extended above head
- Support arms with tape and sandbags; ensure a true lateral.
- Flex legs; secure with tape and sandbags or with retention band across legs and hips; lead shield over pelvic region.

Central Ray: CR ⊥ to IR, centered to **the midcoronal plane**, level of mammillary (nipple) line

SID: Minimum of 50–60 inches (125–150 cm)

Collimation field size: Closely collimate on four sides to outer chest margins.

Respiration: Second full inspiration; if crying, time exposure at full inhalation.

Note: If parental assistance is necessary, have parent hold child's arms overhead, tilting head back with one hand and holding down legs with other hand (provide lead apron and gloves).

kVp Range:				70–85			
	cm	kVp	mA	Time	mAs	SID	Exposure Indicator
S							
M							
L							

Textbook, 11th ed, p. 641

Erect Lateral (With Pigg-O-Stat): Pediatric Chest

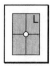

- 8 × 10 inches (18 × 24 cm or 10 × 12 inches 24 × 30 cm) portrait
- Nongrid or grid with systems when it cannot be removed

Position

- With patient remaining in same position as for PA chest, change IR and rotate entire seat and body clamps 90° into a left lateral position; lead shield should be just above iliac crest, ensure that **no rotation** exists.
- Change lead marker to indicate left lateral.

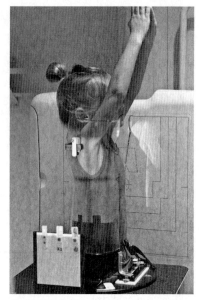

Fig. 1.23 Lateral chest (Pigg-O-Stat, for 5-year-old).

Central Ray: CR ⊥ to IR, centered at level of midthorax, mammillary (nipple) line

SID: 72 inches (180 cm)

Collimation field size: Closely collimate on four sides to outer chest margins.

Respiration: Full inspiration; if crying, time exposure at full inhalation.

| kVp Range: | | | | | 70–85 | |
	cm	kVp	mA	Time	mAs	SID	Exposure Indicator
S							
M							
L							

Textbook, 11th ed, p. 642

PA (AP): Pediatric Chest

Evaluation Criteria
Anatomy Demonstrated
- Entire lungs from apices to costophrenic angles
- Air-filled trachea from T1 down is demonstrated as well as hilum region markings, thymus, heart, and bony thorax.

Position
- Chin elevated sufficiently
- No rotation, equal distance from lateral rib margins to spine
- Full inspiration, visualizes 9 (occasionally 10) posterior ribs above diaphragm

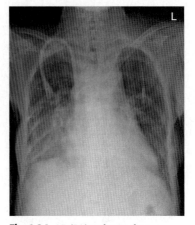

Fig. 1.24 AP (PA) pediatric chest (breathing and voluntary motion is evident, blurred diaphragm).

Exposure
- Optimal image receptor exposure and contrast is sufficient to visualize fine lung markings within lungs.
- Faint outlines of ribs and vertebrae are visible through heart and mediastinal structures.
- No motion, sharp outlines of rib margins, diaphragm and heart shadows

Lateral: Pediatric Chest

Evaluation Criteria

Anatomy Demonstrated
- Entire lungs from apices to costophrenic angles and from sternum anteriorly to posterior ribs

Position
- Chin and arms elevated sufficiently
- No rotation, bilateral posterior ribs and costophrenic angles are superimposed.

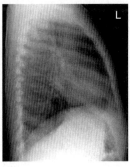

Fig. 1.25 Lateral pediatric chest (DR).

Exposure
- No motion; sharp outline of diaphragm, rib borders, and lung markings
- Optimal image receptor exposure and contrast to faintly visualize ribs and lung markings through heart shadow

Upper Limb

Forearm

Elbow

Pediatric Upper Limb

(R) Routine, (S) Special

Digital Imaging Considerations

The following technical factors are important for all upper limb procedures to maximize image quality:

- 40 inches (100 cm) SID, minimum OID
- Small focal spot
- Nongrid or tabletop (TT)
- Digital imaging requires special attention to **accurate CR and part centering** and **close collimation**.
- Short exposure time
- Immobilization (when needed)
- **Multiple exposures per imaging plate:** Multiple images can be placed on the same IP. When doing so, careful collimation must be used to prevent preexposure or fogging of other images. However, one exposure per IP is recommended.
- Optimal image receptor exposure and contrast with **no motion** to demonstrate soft tissue margins and clear, sharp bony trabecular markings
- **Grid use with digital systems:** Grids are not generally used for upper limb examinations unless the body part (e.g., the shoulder) measures larger than 4 inches (10 cm). Virtual grid technology may eliminate the need for a physical grid.

PA: Fingers

Alternative Routine: Include entire hand on PA finger projection for possible secondary trauma to other parts of hand (see PA Hand).

- 8 × 10 inches (18 × 24 cm) portrait
- Nongrid
- Lead masking with multiple exposures on same IR

Position

- Patient seated, elbow flexed 90° with hand and forearm resting on table
- Pronate hand, separate fingers.
- Center and align long axis of affected finger(s) to portion of IR being exposed.

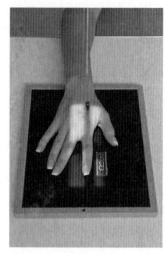

Fig. 2.1 PA—second digit.

Central Ray: CR ⊥, centered to PIP joint

SID: 40 inches (100 cm)

Collimation Field Size: Collimate on four sides to area of interest and distal aspect of metacarpal.

	cm	kVp	mA	Time	mAs	SID	Exposure Indicator
kVp Range:					55–65		
S							
M							
L							

Textbook, 11th ed, p. 138

PA Oblique: Fingers

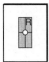

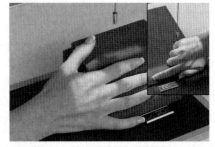

- 8 × 10 inches
  (18 × 24 cm)
  portrait
- Nongrid
- Lead masking with
  multiple exposures
  on same IR

Fig. 2.2 PA oblique, second digit (parallel to IR). *Inset:* Minimized OID.

Position

- Patient seated, hand on table, elbow flexed 90° with hand and forearm resting on table
- Align fingers to long axis of portion of IR being exposed.
- Rotate hand 45° medially or laterally (dependent of digit examined), resting against 45° angle support sponge.
- Separate fingers; ensure that affected finger(s) is (are) parallel to IR.

Central Ray: CR ⊥, centered to PIP joint

SID: 40 inches (100 cm)

Collimation Field Size: Collimate on four sides to area of affected finger(s) and distal aspect of metacarpal.

	cm	kVp	mA	Time	mAs	SID	Exposure Indicator
kVp Range:				55–65			
S							
M							
L							

Textbook, 11th ed, p. 139

PA: Fingers

Evaluation Criteria
Anatomy Demonstrated
- Distal phalanx to distal metacarpal and associated joints

Position
- Long axis of finger parallel to IR with joints open
- No rotation of fingers with symmetric appearance of shafts
- The amount of tissue on each side of the phalanges should appear equal.

Exposure
- Optimal image receptor exposure and contrast; no motion
- Soft tissue margins and clear, sharp bony trabeculation clearly demonstrated

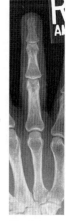

Fig. 2.3 PA finger.

PA Oblique: Fingers

Evaluation Criteria
Anatomy Demonstrated
- Oblique view of distal, middle and proximal phalanx to distal metacarpal and associated joints

Position
- Interphalangeal and MCP joints open
- View of finger being examined should be 45° oblique.
- No superimposition of adjacent digits

Exposure
- Optimal image receptor exposure and contrast; no motion
- Soft tissue margins and clear, sharp bony trabeculation clearly demonstrated; no motion

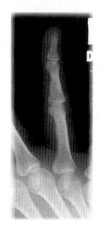

Fig. 2.4 PA oblique finger.

Mediolateral and Lateromedial: Fingers

- 8 × 10 inches (18 × 24 cm) portrait
- Nongrid
- Lead masking with multiple exposures on same IR

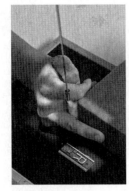

Fig. 2.5 Lateromedial fourth digit.

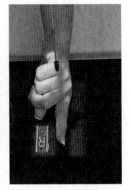

Fig. 2.6 Mediolateral second digit (digit parallel to IR).

Position

Patient seated, hand on table with elbow flexed about 90° with hand and wrist resting on IR and fingers extended

- Hand in lateral position, thumb side up for third to fifth digits, thumb side down for second digit
- Align and center finger to long axis of IR and to CR.
- Use sponge or other radiolucent device to support finger and prevent motion. Flex unaffected fingers.

Central Ray: CR ⊥, centered to PIP joint

SID: 40 inches (100 cm)

Collimation Field Size: Collimate on four sides to affected finger and distal aspect of metacarpal.

	cm	kVp	mA	Time	mAs	SID	Exposure Indicator
kVp Range:				55–65			
S							
M							
L							

Textbook, 11th ed, p. 140

AP: Thumb

- 8 × 10 inches (18 × 24 cm) portrait
- Nongrid
- Lead masking with multiple exposures on same IR

Position

- With patient seated at the end of the table, hand rotated internally to supinate thumb, bring the posterior surface of thumb in direct contact with IR.

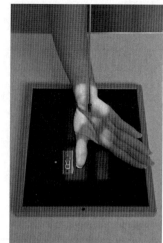

Fig. 2.7 AP thumb—CR to first MP joint.

- Immobilize other fingers with tape to isolate thumb if necessary.
- Align thumb to long axis of portion of IR being exposed.

Central Ray: CR ⊥, centered to first MCP joint

SID: 40 inches (100 cm)

Collimation Field Size: Collimate closely to area of thumb (include entire first metacarpal extending to carpals).

	cm	kVp	mA	Time	mAs	SID	Exposure Indicator
S							
M							
L							

kVp Range: 55–65

Textbook, 11th ed, p. 141

Lateral: Fingers

Evaluation Criteria
Anatomy Demonstrated
- Lateral views of distal, middle, and proximal phalanges; distal metacarpal and associated joints visible

Position
- True lateral position: Joints are open and concave appearance of anterior surfaces of shaft of phalanges

Exposure
- Optimal density (brightness) and contrast; no motion
- Soft tissue margins and clear, sharp bony trabeculation clearly demonstrated

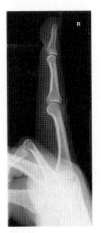

Fig. 2.8 Lateral finger.

AP: Thumb

Evaluation Criteria
Anatomy Demonstrated
- Distal and proximal phalanges, first metacarpal, trapezium, and associated joints are visible

Position
- Long axis of thumb should be aligned with side border of IR
- No rotation of thumb with symmetric appearance of shafts
- Interphalangeal joint should appear open, indicating that thumb was fully extended and correct CR location was used.
- CR and center of collimation field should be at the **first MCP joint**.

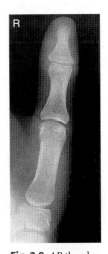

Fig. 2.9 AP thumb.

Exposure
- Optimal image receptor exposure and contrast; no motion
- Soft tissue margins and clear, sharp bony trabeculation clearly demonstrated

PA Oblique: Thumb

- 8 × 10 inches (18 × 24 cm) portrait
- Nongrid
- Lead masking with multiple exposures on same IR

Position
- Patient seated at the end of the table, hand resting on IR, elbow flexed
- Abduct thumb slightly with palmar surface of hand in contact with IR. (This action naturally places thumb in a 45° oblique position.)

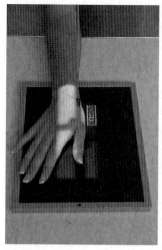

Fig. 2.10 PA oblique thumb, CR to first MCP joint.

- Align long axis of thumb with long axis of IR.

Central Ray: CR ⊥, centered to first MCP joint

SID: 40 inches (100 cm)

Collimation Field Size: Collimate on four sides to thumb, ensuring that **all of first metacarpal and trapezium is included**.

	cm	kVp	mA	Time	mAs	SID	Exposure Indicator
S							
M							
L							

kVp Range: 55–65

Textbook, 11th ed, p. 142

Lateral: Thumb

- 8 × 10 inches (18 × 24 cm) portrait
- Nongrid
- Lead masking with multiple exposures on same IR

Position

- Patient seated at end of table, elbow flexed 90° with hand resting on IR, palm down
- With hand pronated and thumb abducted, with fingers and hand slightly arched, rotate hand medially until thumb is in true lateral position.

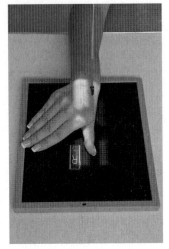

Fig. 2.11 Lateral thumb, CR to first MCP joint.

- Align thumb to long axis of portion of IR being exposed.

Central Ray: CR ⊥, centered to first MCP joint

SID: 40 inches (100 cm)

Collimation Field Size: Collimate on four sides to thumb area. (Remember that first metacarpal and trapezium must be within the field of view.)

kVp Range:					55–65	
	cm	kVp	mA	Time	mAs	SID	Exposure Indicator
S							
M							
L							

Textbook, 11th ed, p. 143

PA Oblique: Thumb

Evaluation Criteria

Anatomy Demonstrated
- Distal and proximal phalanges, first metacarpal, trapezium, and associated joints are visualized in a 45° oblique position.

Position
- Long axis of thumb should be aligned with side border of IR.
- Interphalangeal and metacarpophalangeal joints should appear open if the phalanges are parallel to the IR and if the CR location is correct.
- CR and center of collimation field should be at **first MCP joint**.

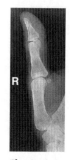

Fig. 2.12 PA oblique thumb.

Exposure
- Optimal image receptor exposure and contrast; no motion
- Soft tissue margins and clear, sharp bony trabeculation clearly demonstrated

---

Lateral: Thumb

Evaluation Criteria

Anatomy Demonstrated
- Distal and proximal phalanges, first metacarpal, trapezium (superimposed), and associated joints are visualized in the lateral position.

Position
- Long axis of thumb should be aligned with side border of IR.
- Thumb should be in a true lateral position.
- Interphalangeal and metacarpophalangeal joints should appear open.
- CR and center of collimation field should be at the **first MCP joint**.

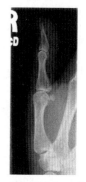

Fig. 2.13 Lateral thumb.

Exposure
- Optimal density (brightness) and contrast; no motion
- Soft tissue margins and clear, sharp bony trabeculation clearly demonstrated

AP Axial: Thumb
Modified Robert Method

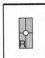

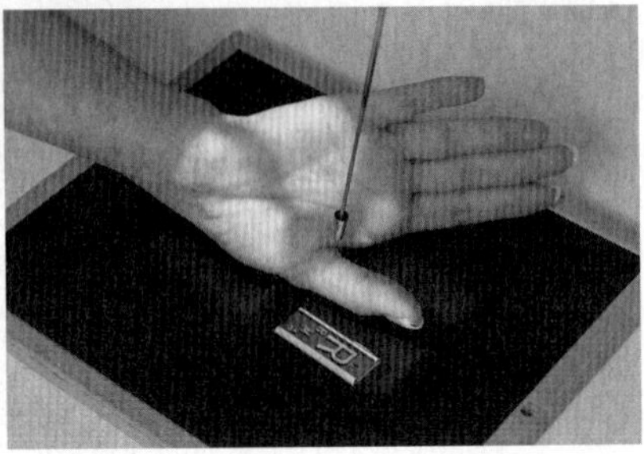

Note: This is a special projection to better demonstrate the **first carpometacarpal joint** region.

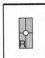

Fig. 2.14 AP axial thumb for first CMC joint (CR 15° proximally).

- 8 × 10 inches (18 × 24 cm) portrait
- Nongrid
- Lead masking with multiple exposures on same IR

Position
- Patient seated, hand and arm extended, and arm rotated internally until posterior aspect of thumb rests on IR
- Place thumb in center of IR, parallel to side border of IR
- Extend fingers

Central Ray: CR angled 10–15° proximally (toward wrist), centered to first CMC joint; the **Lewis modification**—CR angle 10° to 15° proximal to MCP

SID: 40 inches (100 cm)

Collimation Field Size: Collimate on four sides to area of thumb and first CMC joint.

	cm	kVp	mA	Time	mAs	SID	Exposure Indicator
S							
M							
L							

kVp Range: 55–65

Textbook, 11th ed, p. 144

PA: Hand

- 10 × 12 inches (18 × 24 cm) portrait
- Nongrid

Position

- Patient seated, hand on table, elbow flexed
- Hand fully pronated; digits slightly separated
- Align long axis of hand and forearm with long axis of IR.

Central Ray: CR ⊥, centered to third MCP joint

SID: 40 inches (100 cm)

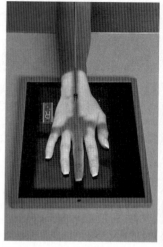

Fig. 2.15 PA hand.

Collimation Field Size: Collimate on four sides to outer margins of hand and wrist.

	cm	kVp	mA	Time	mAs	SID	Exposure Indicator
S							
M							
L							

kVp Range: 55–65

Textbook, 11th ed, p. 146

AP Axial: Thumb
Modified Robert Method

Evaluation Criteria
Anatomy Demonstrated
- AP projection of the thumb and first CMC joint are visible without superimposition.
- Base of first metacarpal and trapezium should be well visualized.

Position
- Long axis of thumb should be aligned with side border of IR.
- **No rotation**
- First CMC and MCP joints should appear open.
- CR and center of collimation field should be at **first CMC joint**.

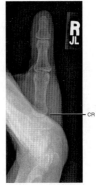

Fig. 2.16 AP axial thumb (modified Robert).

Exposure
- Optimal image receptor exposure and contrast; no motion
- Soft tissue margins and clear, sharp bony trabeculation clearly demonstrated

---

PA: Hand

Evaluation Criteria
Anatomy Demonstrated
- PA projection of entire hand and wrist and about 1 inch (2.5 cm) of distal forearm are visible.
- PA projection of hand demonstrates oblique view of the thumb.

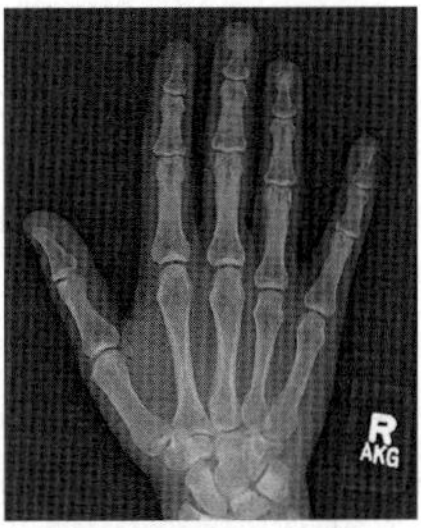

Position
- Long axis of hand and wrist aligned with long axis of IR

Fig. 2.17 PA hand.

- **No rotation** of hand. Digits should be separated slightly with soft tissues not overlapping.
- MCP and IP joints should appear open, indicating correct CR location and that hand was fully pronated.
- CR and center of collimation field should be to **third MCP joint**.

Exposure
- Optimal image receptor exposure and contrast; no motion
- Soft tissue margins and clear, sharp bony trabeculation clearly demonstrated

PA Oblique: Hand

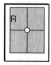

- 10 × 12 inches (24 × 30 cm) portrait
- Nongrid

Position
- Patient seated, hand and forearm extended, elbow flexed
- Rotate entire hand and wrist laterally 45°, support with wedge step sponge; align hand and wrist to IR.
- Ensure that all digits are slightly separated and parallel to IR.

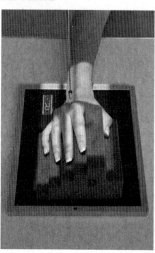

Fig. 2.18 PA oblique hand (digits parallel to IR).

Central Ray: CR ⊥, centered to third MCP joint
SID: 40 inches (100 cm)
Collimation Field Size: Collimate on four sides to hand and wrist.

	cm	kVp	mA	Time	mAs	SID	Exposure Indicator
S							
M							
L							

kVp Range: 55–65

Textbook, 11th ed, p. 147

"Fan" Lateral and Lateral in Extension: Hand

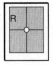

- 10 × 12 inches (24 × 30 cm) portrait
- Nongrid
- Accessory— foam step support

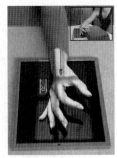

Fig. 2.19 "Fan" lateral hand (digits not superimposed).

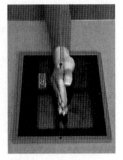

Fig. 2.20 Alternative: lateral in extension (for possible foreign body and metacarpal injury).

2

Upper Limb

Position

- Patient seated, with hand and forearm extended
- Rotate hand and wrist into lateral position, thumb side up, digits separated and spread into "fan" position and supported by radiolucent step sponge or similar-type support. (Ensure true lateral of metacarpals.)

Central Ray: CR ⊥, centered to second MCP joint
SID: 40 inches (100 cm)
Collimation Field Size: Collimate on four sides to outer margins of hand and wrist.

	cm	kVp	mA	Time	mAs	SID	Exposure Indicator
kVp Range:					55–65		
S							
M							
L							

Textbook, 11th ed, pp. 148 and 149

Evaluation Criteria
Anatomy Demonstrated
• Oblique projection of the entire hand and wrist and about 1 inch (2.5 cm) of distal forearm are visible.

Position
• Long axis of hand and wrist should be aligned with IR.
• 45° oblique is evidenced by the following: midshafts of metacarpals should not overlap; some overlap of distal heads of third, fourth, and fifth metacarpals but no overlap of distal second and third metacarpals should occur.

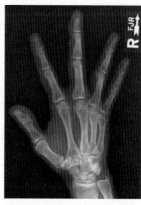

Fig. 2.21 PA oblique hand (digits parallel).

• MCP and IP joints are open without foreshortening of midphalanges or distal phalanges.
• CR and center of collimation field should be at third MCP joint.

Exposure
• Optimal image receptor exposure and contrast; no motion
• Soft tissue margins and clear, sharp bony trabeculation clearly demonstrated

"Fan" Lateral: Hand

Evaluation Criteria

Anatomy Demonstrated

- Entire hand and wrist and about 1 inch (2.5 cm) of distal forearm are visible.

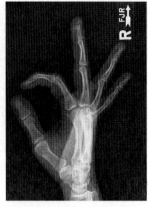

Fig. 2.22 "Fan" lateral hand.

Position

- Long axis of hand and wrist should be aligned with long axis of IR.
- Fingers should appear equally separated, with phalanges in lateral position and joint spaces open.
- Thumb should appear in slightly oblique position completely free of superimposition, with joint spaces open.
- Hand and wrist should be in a true lateral position.
- CR and center of collimation field should be at **second MCP joint**.

Exposure

- Optimal image receptor exposure and contrast; no motion
- Soft tissue margins and clear, sharp bony trabeculation clearly demonstrated

Upper Limb

AP Axial Projection: Hand
Brewerton method

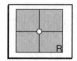

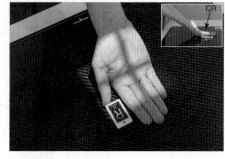

Fig. 2.23 AP axial (Brewerton method).

- 10 × 12 inches (24 × 30 cm) portrait or 14 × 17 (35 × 43 cm) bilateral study, landscape
- Nongrid

Position
- Patient seated, with hand supinated and flexed
- From this position, keeping fingers in contact with the IR, flex the hand to create a 65° angle between the dorsum of hand and IR.
- Extend fingers and ensure they are relaxed, slightly separated, and parallel to IR.
- Abduct thumb to avoid superimposition.

Central Ray: CR angled 15° proximally, toward ulna, directed to the **third MCP joint**

SID: 40 inches (100 cm)

Collimation Field Size: Collimate on four sides to outer margins of hand and wrist.

	cm	kVp	mA	Time	mAs	SID	Exposure Indicator
S							
M							
L							

kVp Range: 55–65

Textbook, 11th ed, p. 150

AP Axial Projection: Hand
Brewerton Method

Evaluation Criteria

Anatomy Demonstrated

- Entire hand from the carpal area to the tips of digits is visible. This projection is intended for the assessment for early signs of rheumatoid arthritis in the MCP, PIP, and DIP joints.

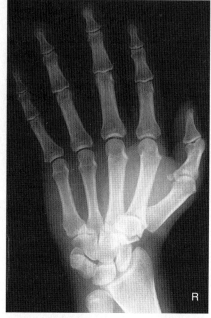

Fig. 2.24 AP axial (Brewerton method). (From Wilson DJ et al: *Musculoskeletal imaging*, ed 2, Philadelphia, 2015, Elsevier.)

Position

- Second through fifth MCP joints should be open and visible with no superimposition of the palmer soft tissue; thumb free of superimposition with second through fifth digits.
- Midshafts of second through fifth metacarpals and phalanges should not overlap or be rotated.
- CR and center of collimation field should be **at the third MCP joint**.

Exposure

- Optimal image receptor exposure and contrast; no motion
- Soft tissue margins and clear, sharp bony trabeculation with MCP joints clearly demonstrated

PA: Wrist

- 8 × 10 inches (18 × 24 cm) portrait
- Nongrid
- Lead masking with multiple exposures on same IR

Position
- Patient seated, arm on table with hand and forearm extended
- Lower shoulder so that shoulder, elbow, and wrist are on same horizontal plane.
- Align and center long axis of hand and wrist parallel to edge of IR.
- Hand pronated, fingers flexed, and hand arched slightly to place wrist and carpal area in close contact with IR

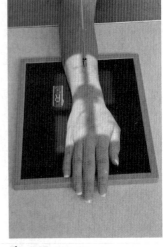

Fig. 2.25 PA wrist.

Central Ray: CR ⊥, centered to midcarpals
SID: 40 inches (100 cm)
Collimation Field Size: Collimate to wrist on all four sides.

	cm	kVp	mA	Time	mAs	SID	Exposure Indicator
S							
M							
L							

kVp Range: 55–65

Textbook, 11th ed, p. 151

PA Oblique: Wrist

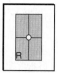

- 8 × 10 inches (18 × 24 cm) portrait
- Nongrid
- Lead masking with multiple exposures on same IR

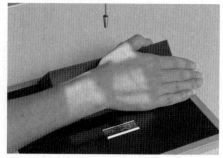

Fig. 2.26 45° PA oblique wrist (with support).

Position

- Patient seated, arm on table with hand and forearm extended
- Align and center hand and wrist to IR.
- Rotate hand and wrist laterally into 45° oblique position.
- Flex fingers to support hand in this position, or use 45° sponge.

Central Ray: CR ⊥, centered to midcarpals

SID: 40 inches (100 cm)

Collimation Field Size: Collimate to wrist on four sides.

	cm	kVp	mA	Time	mAs	SID	Exposure Indicator
kVp Range:					60–70		
S							
M							
L							

Textbook, 11th ed, p. 152

PA: Wrist

Evaluation Criteria
Anatomy Demonstrated

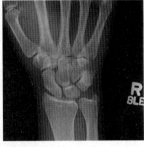

Fig. 2.27 PA wrist.

- Midmetacarpals and proximal metacarpals; carpals; distal radius, ulna, and associated joints and pertinent soft tissues of the wrist joint, such as fat pads and fat stripes, are visible.
- All the intercarpal spaces do not appear open because of irregular shapes that result in overlapping.

Position
- True PA is evidenced by symmetry of proximal metacarpals.
- Separation of the distal radius and ulna
- CR and center of collimation field should be to the **midcarpal area**.

Exposure
- Optimal image receptor exposure and contrast; no motion
- Soft tissue margins and clear, sharp bony trabeculation of carpals clearly demonstrated

PA Oblique: Wrist

Evaluation Criteria
Anatomy Demonstrated

- Distal radius, ulna, carpals, and at least to midmetacarpals; carpals; distal radius, ulna, and associated joints are visible. Trapezium and scaphoid should be well visualized, with only slight superimposition of other carpals on their medial aspects.

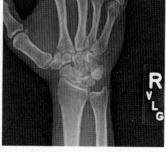

Fig. 2.28 PA oblique wrist.

Position
- Long axis of hand, wrist, and forearm aligned to IR
- 45° oblique of wrist
- CR and center of collimation field should be to **midcarpal area**.

Exposure
- Optimal image receptor exposure and contrast; no motion
- Soft tissue margins and clear, sharp bony trabeculation of carpals clearly demonstrated

Lateral: Wrist

- 8 × 10 inches (18 × 24 cm) portrait
- Nongrid
- Lead masking with multiple exposures on same IR

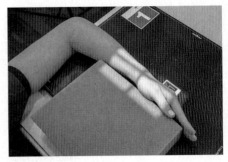

Fig. 2.29 Lateral wrist.

Position

- Patient seated, arm and forearm on table, shoulder dropped to place humerus, forearm, and wrist on same horizontal plane
- Align and center hand and wrist parallel to edge of IR.
- Place hand and wrist into a true lateral position; use support to maintain this position if needed.

Central Ray: CR ⊥, centered to midcarpals

SID: 40 inches (100 cm)

Collimation Field Size: Collimate to wrist on four sides.

kVp Range:					60–70	
	cm	kVp	mA	Time	mAs	SID	Exposure Indicator
S							
M							
L							

Textbook, 11th ed, p. 153

Lateral: Wrist

Evaluation Criteria

Anatomy Demonstrated
- Distal radius and ulna, carpals, and at least the midmetacarpal area

Position
- Long axis of the hand, wrist, and forearm should be aligned with long axis of IR
- True lateral of wrist*
- Ulnar head superimposed distal radius
- CR and center of collimation field should be to **midcarpal region**.

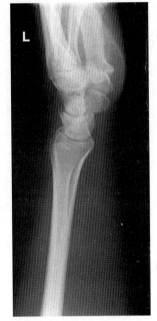

Fig. 2.30 Lateral wrist.

Exposure
- Optimal image receptor exposure and contrast; no motion
- Soft tissue margins and clear, sharp bony trabeculation of carpals clearly demonstrated
- Demonstrate visible fat pads of the wrist and borders of the distal ulna, seen through the superimposed radius.*

---

*To achieve a true lateral of the wrist joint, the wrist may require 10-15 degrees of elevation away from the IR.

PA and PA Axial With Ulnar Deviation: Scaphoid
10°–15° and Modified Stecher Method

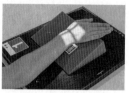

Fig. 2.31 Ulnar deviation, CR 10°–15° angle toward elbow. CR perpendicular to scaphoid.

Warning: If patient has possible wrist trauma, do not attempt this position before a routine wrist series has been completed and evaluated to rule out possible fracture of distal forearm, wrist, or both.

Note: See Chapter 1 in the 11th edition of this textbook for joint movement terminology.

- 8 × 10 inches (18 × 24 cm) portrait
- Nongrid
- Lead masking with multiple exposures on same IR

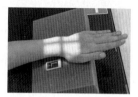

Fig. 2.32 Modified Stecher method. Elevate hand on 20° sponge, CR ⊥ to IR.

Position

- Patient seated with wrist and hand on IR, palm down, and shoulder, elbow, and wrist on the same horizontal plane
- From PA wrist position, gently deviate wrist toward ulnar side as far as the patient can tolerate without lifting or rotating distal forearm.

Central Ray: CR perpendicular to IR. Optional CR angled 10°–15° proximally toward elbow, centered to scaphoid (thumb side of carpal area); if hand placed on 20° sponge, CR ⊥ to IR

Note: A four-projection series with CR at 0°, 10°, 20°, and 30° may be required.

SID: 40 inches (100 cm)

Collimation Field Size: Collimate on four sides to carpal region.

	cm	kVp	mA	Time	mAs	SID	Exposure Indicator
kVp Range:			55–65				
S							
M							
L							

Textbook, 11th ed, pp. 154 and 155

PA and PA Axial With Ulnar Deviation: Scaphoid
10°–15° Ulnar Deviation and Modified Stecher Method

Evaluation Criteria

Anatomy Demonstrated

- Distal radius and ulna, carpals, and proximal metacarpals are visible; no motion.
- Scaphoid demonstrated clearly without foreshortening
- Soft tissue margins and clear, sharp bony trabeculation of scaphoid clearly demonstrated

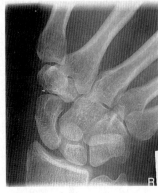

Fig. 2.33 Ulnar deviation with 10°–15° CR angle.

Position

- Long axis of wrist and forearm should be aligned with side border of IR.
- Ulnar deviation evident
- No rotation of wrist
- Multiple CR angles may help to best visualize this area.

Exposure

- Optimal image receptor exposure and contrast; no motion
- Soft tissue margins and clear, sharp bony trabeculation of scaphoid clearly demonstrated

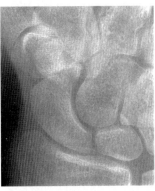

Fig. 2.34 Modified Stecher.

PA With Radial Deviation: Wrist

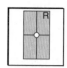

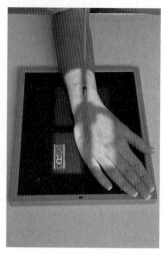

Warning: If patient has possible wrist trauma, do not attempt this position before a routine wrist series has been completed and evaluated to rule out possible fracture of distal forearm or wrist.

Note: See Chapter 1 (pp. 11 to 14) in the 11th edition textbook, for an explanation of wrist joint movement terminology.

- 8 × 10 inches (18 × 24 cm) portrait
- Nongrid
- Lead masking with multiple exposures on same IR

Fig. 2.35 Radial deviation, CR perpendicular. (Demonstrates ulnar side carpals.)

Position

- Patient seated with hand and forearm extended. Drop shoulder so that shoulder, elbow, and wrist are on same horizontal plane.
- From PA wrist position, gently invert wrist toward thumb side as far as patient can tolerate.

Central Ray: CR ⊥ to midcarpal area

SID: 40 inches (100 cm)

Collimation Field Size: Collimate closely to four sides of carpal region.

	cm	kVp	mA	Time	mAs	SID	Exposure Indicator
kVp Range:					55–65		
S							
M							
L							

Textbook, 11th ed, p. 157

PA With Radial Deviation: Wrist

Evaluation Criteria

Anatomy Demonstrated

- Distal radius and ulna, carpals, and proximal metacarpals are visible.
- Ulnar side carpals best visualized

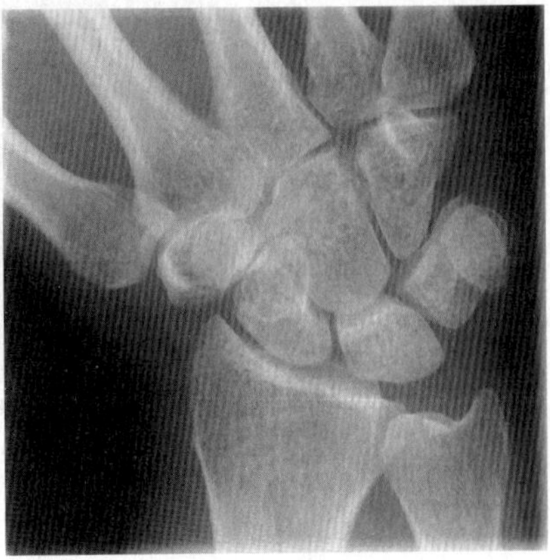

Position

- Long axis of wrist and forearm should be aligned with side border of IR.
- Extreme radial deviation evident
- No rotation of wrist
- CR and center of the collimation field should be to the **midcarpal area**.

Exposure

- Optimal density (brightness) and contrast; no motion
- Soft tissue margins and clear, sharp bony trabeculation of ulnar aspect of carpal region clearly demonstrated

Fig. 2.36 PA wrist—radial deviation.

Bilateral PA Stress ("Clenched" PA) Scaphoid

Clinical indications:

- Possible scaphoid fracture
- Possible scapholunate ligament injury evident by a widening of the lunate from the scaphoid (>3-4 mm)

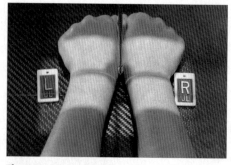

Fig. 2.37 Bilateral PA Stress ("Clenched" PA) Scaphoid.

- Recommended field size—8 × 10 inches (18 × 24 cm), portrait
- Nongrid

Position

- Position wrists as for PA projection—palm down with wrist and hand aligned with center of long axis of IR.
- Ensure there is no rotation of hands and wrists
- Index fingers are opposed tightly to each other
- Ask patient to clench fists equally (Fig. 2.37)

Central Ray: CR perpendicular to IR directed to midpoint between both carpal regions

SID: 40 inches (100 cm)

Collimation Field Size: Collimate on four sides to bilateral carpal region.

kVp Range:					55–65		
	cm	kVp	mA	Time	mAs	SID	Exposure Indicator
S							
M							
L							

Textbook, 11th ed, p. 156

Bilateral PA Stress ("Clenched" PA)

Evaluation Criteria
Anatomy Demonstrated
- Distal radius and ulna, carpals, and proximal metacarpals are visible.
- Carpals are visible, with adjacent interspaces more open on the medial (ulnar) side of the wrist.

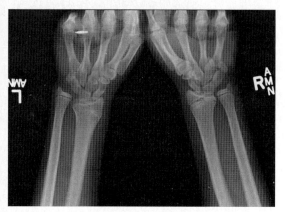

Fig. 2.38 Bilateral PA Stress ("Clenched" PA). (Courtesy of Joshua M. Abzug, MD. From Abzug JM et al: *Pediatric hand therapy*, Philadelphia, 2020, Elsevier.)

Position
- Long axis of the forearm is aligned with the side border of IR
- **No rotation** of the wrist is evidenced by the appearance of the distal radius and ulna.
- CR and center of the collimation field should be to the **midcarpal area**.

Exposure
- Optimal image receptor exposure and contrast with **no motion** visualize the carpal borders and clear, sharp bony trabecular markings.

Tangential Inferosuperior: Wrist (Carpal Canal)
Gaynor-Hart Method

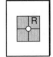

Warning: This position is sometimes called the "carpal tunnel view." If the patient has possible wrist trauma, do *not* attempt this position before a routine wrist series has been completed and evaluated to rule out possible fracture of the distal forearm or wrist.

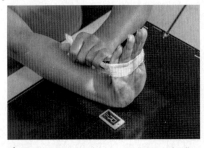

Fig. 2.39 Tangential (Gaynor-Hart method) projection (CR 25°–30° to long axis of hand).

- 8 × 10 inches (18 × 24 cm) portrait
- Nongrid
- Lead masking with multiple exposures on same IR

Position
- Patient seated, wrist and hand on IR, palm down
- Align hand and wrist with long axis of the IR.
- Hyperextend (dorsiflex) wrist as far as patient can tolerate with patient using other hand to hold fingers back, or tape may be used.
- Rotate hand and wrist slightly internally—toward radius (≈10°).
- Work quickly, as this may be painful for patient.

Central Ray: CR angled 25°–30° proximally to long axis of the palmar surface of hand, centered to ≈1 inch (2–3 cm) distal to base of third metacarpal

SID: 40 inches (100 cm)

Collimation Field Size: Collimate on four sides to carpal region.

	cm	kVp	mA	Time	mAs	SID	Exposure Indicator
kVp Range:					**55–65**		
S							
M							
L							

Textbook, 11th ed, p. 158

Tangential Inferosuperior: Wrist (Carpal Canal)
Gaynor-Hart Method

Evaluation Criteria

Anatomy Demonstrated
- Carpal sulcus demonstrated in a tunnel-like, arched arrangement

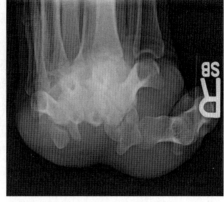

Fig. 2.40 Tangential (Gaynor-Hart).

Position
- Pisiform and the hamular process separated (if not, wrist was not rotated 10° toward radius)
- Capitate, scaphoid/trapezium in profile
- CR and center of collimation field should be to **midpoint of the carpal canal**.

Exposure
- Optimal image receptor exposure and contrast; no motion
- Soft tissue margins and clear, sharp bony trabeculation of carpal canal clearly demonstrated

AP: Forearm

- 14 × 17 inches (35 × 43 cm) portrait; 10 × 12 inches (24 × 30 cm) portrait for smaller patients
- Nongrid

Position

- Patient seated, with hand and arm extended and hand supinated
- Drop shoulder to place entire upper limb on same horizontal plane.

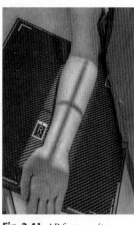

Fig. 2.41 AP forearm (to include both joints).

- Align and center forearm to long axis of IR, ensuring that both wrist and elbow joints are included (use as large an IR as required to include both wrist and elbow joints).
- Have patient lean laterally as needed for a true AP of forearm.

Central Ray: CR ⊥, centered to midpoint of forearm

SID: 40 inches (100 cm)

Collimation Field Size: Collimate on four sides. Include a minimum of 1 inch (2.5 cm) beyond both wrist and elbow joints.

	cm	kVp	mA	Time	mAs	SID	Exposure Indicator
S							
M							
L							

kVp Range: 65–75

Textbook, 11th ed, p. 161

Lateromedial: Forearm

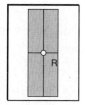

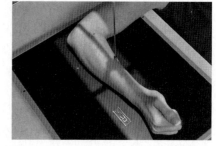

Fig. 2.42 Lateral forearm (to include both joints).

- 14 × 17 inches (35 × 43 cm) portrait or 10 × 12 inches (24 × 30 cm) portrait for smaller patients
- Nongrid

Position

- Patient seated with elbow flexed 90°
- Drop shoulder to place entire upper limb on same horizontal plane.
- Rotate hand and wrist into true lateral position (distal radius and ulna should be directly superimposed).
- Ensure that both wrist and elbow joints are included unless contraindicated.

Central Ray: CR ⊥, centered to midpoint of forearm
SID: 40 inches (100 cm)
Collimation Field Size: Collimate on four sides. Include a minimum of 1 inch (2.5 cm) beyond both wrist and elbow joints.

kVp Range:					65–75		
	cm	kVp	mA	Time	mAs	SID	Exposure Indicator
S							
M							
L							

Textbook, 11th ed, p. 162

AP: Forearm

Evaluation Criteria

Anatomy Demonstrated
- Entire radius and ulna with a minimum of proximal row carpals and distal humerus and pertinent soft tissues, such as fat pads and stripes of the wrist and elbow joints

Position
- Long axis of forearm should be aligned with long axis of IR.
- No rotation of forearm, as evidenced by slight superimposition of proximal radius/ulna
- Humeral epicondyles in profile
- CR and center of collimation field should be to the **approximate midpoint of the radius and ulna**.

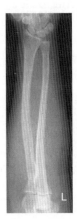

Fig. 2.43 AP forearm.

Exposure
- Optimal image receptor exposure and contrast; no motion
- Soft tissue margins and clear, sharp bony trabeculation clearly demonstrated

Lateromedial: Forearm

Evaluation Criteria
Anatomy Demonstrated
- Entire radius and ulna demonstrated, proximal row of carpal bones, elbow, and distal end of the humerus are visible as well as pertinent soft tissue, such as fat pads and stripes of the wrist and elbow joints.

Position
- Long axis of forearm should be aligned with long axis of IR.
- Elbow should be flexed 90° for true lateral position.
- **No rotation**, as evidenced by head of ulna being superimposed over the radius, and humeral epicondyles should be superimposed.
- Radial head should superimpose coronoid process, with radial tuberosity demonstrated.
- CR and center of collimation field should be to **midpoint of the radius and ulna**.

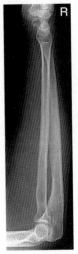

Fig. 2.44
Lateral forearm.

Exposure
- Optimal image receptor exposure and contrast; no motion
- Soft tissue margins and clear, sharp bony trabeculation of carpal canal clearly demonstrated, and fat pads and stripes of the wrist and elbow joints

AP: Elbow
Fully and Partially Extended

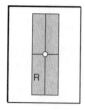

- 10 × 12 inches (24 × 30 cm) portrait
- Nongrid

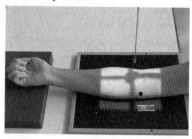

Fig. 2.45 AP, fully extended.

Position
- Patient seated, elbow extended and hand supinated
- Lean laterally as needed for true AP (palpate epicondyles)
- If elbow cannot be fully extended, obtain two AP projections, as shown (Figs. 2.46 and 2.47), with CR perpendicular to distal humerus on one and perpendicular to proximal forearm on another.

Central Ray: CR ⊥, centered to midelbow joint

SID: 40 inches (100 cm)

Collimation Field Size: Collimate on four sides to area of interest.

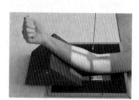

Fig. 2.46 CR, ⊥ to humerus.

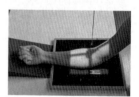

Fig. 2.47 CR ⊥ to forearm.

	cm	kVp	mA	Time	mAs	SID	Exposure Indicator
kVp Range:					65–75		
S							
M							
L							

Textbook, 11th ed, pp. 163 and 164

AP: Elbow
Fully Extended

Evaluation Criteria
Anatomy Demonstrated
- Distal humerus, elbow joint space, and proximal radius and ulna

Position
- Long axis of arm should be aligned with long axis of IR.
- No rotation, as evidenced by slight superimposition of proximal radius/ulna
- Humeral epicondyles in profile
- CR and center of collimation field should be to the midelbow joint.

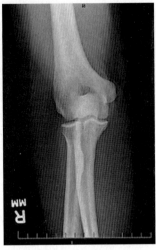

Fig. 2.48 AP elbow fully extended.

Exposure
- Optimal image receptor exposure and contrast; no motion
- Soft tissue margins and clear, sharp bony trabeculation of elbow clearly demonstrated

AP: Elbow
Partially Flexed

Evaluation Criteria
Anatomy Demonstrated

- Distal ⅓ of humerus; best visualized on "humerus parallel" projection
- Proximal ⅓ of forearm; best visualized on "forearm parallel" projection

Position

- Long axis of arm should be aligned with side border of IR.
- No rotation, as evidenced by slight superimposition of proximal radius/ulna
- Humeral epicondyles in profile
- CR and center of collimation field should be to the **midelbow joint**.

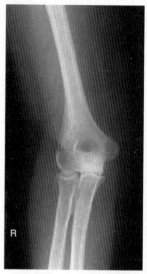

Fig. 2.49 Humerus parallel to IR.

Exposure

- Optimal image receptor exposure and contrast; no motion
- Distal humerus, including epicondyles, is demonstrated with sufficient density on "humerus parallel" projection Fig. 2.49.
- On "forearm parallel" projection, proximal radius and ulna should be well visualized to allow visualization of both soft tissue and bony detail Fig. 2.50.
- Soft tissue and clear, sharp bony trabeculation clearly demonstrated

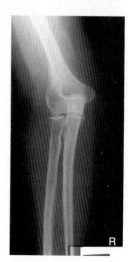

Fig. 2.50 Forearm parallel to IR.

AP Oblique (Medial and Lateral): Elbow

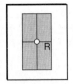

The **medial (internal) oblique** best visualizes the coronoid process. The **lateral (external) oblique** best visualizes the radial head and neck (most common oblique projection):

- 10 × 12 inches (24 × 30 cm) portrait
- Nongrid

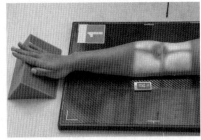

Fig. 2.51 Medial (internal) oblique (45°).

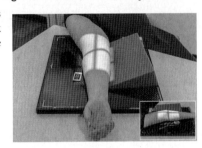

Fig. 2.52 Lateral (external) oblique (40°–45°).

Position
Medial Oblique:
- Elbow extended; hand pronated
- Palpate epicondyles to check for 45° internal rotation

Lateral Oblique: Similar position, except supinate hand and rotate elbow 40°–45° externally; more difficult for patient; lean entire upper body laterally, as needed. Palpate epicondyles to check for 45° external rotation.

Central Ray: CR ⊥, centered to midelbow joint

SID: 40 inches (100 cm)

Collimation Field Size: Collimate on four sides to area of interest.

	cm	kVp	mA	Time	mAs	SID	Exposure Indicator
kVp Range:				65–75			
S							
M							
L							

Textbook, 11th ed, pp. 166 and 168

Upper Limb

AP Oblique (Medial): Elbow

Evaluation Criteria

Anatomy Demonstrated
- Proximal radius and ulna
- Medial epicondyle and trochlea

Position
- Coronoid process in profile
- Radial head/neck superimposed over ulna

Exposure
- Optimal image receptor exposure and contrast soft tissue margins and clear, sharp bony trabeculation clearly demonstrated

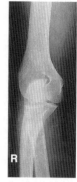

Fig. 2.53 Medial (internal) oblique elbow.

AP Oblique (Lateral): Elbow

Evaluation Criteria

Anatomy Demonstrated
- Oblique projection of distal humerus, proximal radius, and ulna
- Lateral epicondyle and capitulum

Position
- Long axis of arm should be aligned with side border of IR.
- Correct 45° lateral oblique should allow visualization of radial head, neck, and tuberosity free of superimposition by ulna.
- Humeral epicondyles and capitulum should be in profile.
- CR and center of collimation field should be to **midelbow joint**.

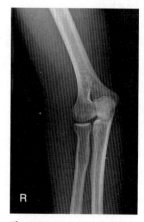

Fig. 2.54 Lateral (external) oblique elbow.

Exposure
- Optimal image receptor exposure and contrast; no motion
- Soft tissue margins and clear, sharp bony trabeculation demonstrated

Lateromedial: Elbow

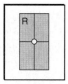

- 10 × 12 inches (24 × 30 cm) portrait
- Nongrid

Position
- Patient seated, elbow flexed 90°, shoulder dropped as needed to rest forearm and humerus flat on table and IR
- Align long axis of forearm with long axis of IR.

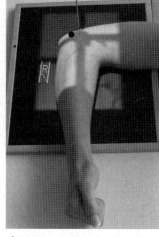

Fig. 2.55 Lateral—elbow flexed 90°.

- Center elbow joint to CR and to center of IR, with forearm aligned parallel to edge of cassette.
- Place hand and wrist in a true lateral position, thumb side up.

Central Ray: CR ⊥, centered to midelbow joint
SID: 40 inches (100 cm)
Collimation Field Size: Collimate on four sides.

	cm	kVp	mA	Time	mAs	SID	Exposure Indicator
kVp Range:				65–75			
S							
M							
L							

Textbook, 11th ed, p. 169

Lateromedial: Elbow

Evaluation Criteria

Anatomy Demonstrated

- Lateral projection of proximal radius/ulna and distal humerus, olecranon process, and soft tissues and fat pads of the elbow joint are visible.

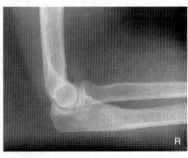

Fig. 2.56 Lateromedial elbow.

Position

- Long axis of the forearm should be aligned with long axis of IR, with the elbow joint flexed 90°.
- About one-half of radial head should be superimposed by the coronoid process, and the olecranon process should be visualized in profile.
- True lateral should occur, as indicated by three concentric arcs of the trochlear sulcus, double ridges of the capitulum and trochlea, and the trochlear notch of the ulna.
- Superimposition of the humeral epicondyles occurs.
- CR and center of collimation field should be **midpoint of the elbow joint**.

Exposure

- Optimal image receptor exposure and contrast; no motion
- Soft tissue margins and clear, sharp bony trabeculation clearly demonstrated as well as soft tissue margins of the anterior and posterior fat pads

Axial Lateromedial and Mediolateral: Elbow (Trauma)
Coyle Method

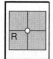

Special views will demonstrate the **radial head** and **coronoid process**.

- 10 × 12 inches (24 × 30 cm) portrait
- Nongrid

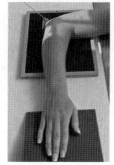

Fig. 2.57 For radial head and neck, elbow flexed 90°.

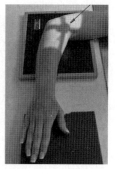

Fig. 2.58 For coronoid process, elbow flexed 80°.

Position and Central Ray
Radial Head
- Patient seated or supine, elbow flexed **90°** if possible, hand pronated
- Angle CR 45° toward shoulder, centered to radial head (CR to enter at midelbow joint)

Coronoid Process
- Elbow flexed **only 80°** from extended position, with hand pronated
- Angle CR 45° away from shoulder, centered to enter at mid-elbow joint)

SID: 40 inches (100 cm)

Collimation Field Size: Collimate on four sides to area of interest.

	cm	kVp	mA	Time	mAs	SID	Exposure Indicator
S							
M							
L							

kVp Range: 70–80

Textbook, 11th ed, p. 170

Axial Lateromedial and Mediolateral: Elbow (Trauma)
Coyle Method

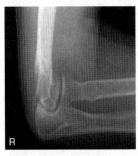

Fig. 2.59 Trauma axial lateral elbow (for radial head, neck, and capitulum).

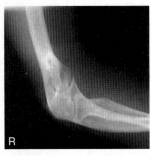

Fig. 2.60 Trauma axial lateral elbow (for coronoid process and trochlea).

Evaluation Criteria

Anatomy Demonstrated and Position—Radial Head (CR 45° Toward Shoulder: Lateromedial Projection)

- Radial head, neck, and capitulum projected away from proximal ulna; elbow flexed **90°**

Anatomy Demonstrated and Position—Coronoid Process (CR 45° Away From Shoulder: Mediolateral Projection)

- Coronoid process and trochlea demonstrated
- Coronoid process in profile, elbow flexed **80°** (flexion of more than 80° will obscure coronoid process)

Exposure

- Optimal image receptor exposure and contrast; no motion
- Soft tissue margins and clear, sharp bony trabeculation clearly demonstrated

AP: Upper Limb (Pediatric)

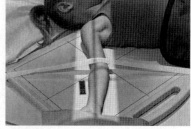

With possible trauma, handle limb very gently with minimal movement. Obtain a single exposure to rule out

Fig. 2.61 AP—upper limb.

gross fractures before additional images are taken.
- IR size determined by patient age and size
- Nongrid

Position
- Immobilize with clear flexible-type retention band and sandbags, or with tape when necessary.
- Use the supine position, arm abducted away from body.
- Include entire limb unless a specific joint or bone is indicated.
- Supinate hand and forearm into the AP position (with hand and fingers extended.
- Use parental assistance only if necessary; provide lead gloves and apron.

Central Ray: CR ⊥, centered to midlimb
SID: 40 inches (100 cm)
Collimation Field Size: Collimate on four sides to area of interest.

	cm	kVp	mA	Time	mAs	SID	Exposure Indicator
kVp Range:				50–60			
S							
M							
L							

Textbook, 11th ed, p. 643

 2

Upper Limb

Latheral: Upper Limb (Pediatric)

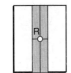

- IR size determined by patient age and size
- Nongrid

Position

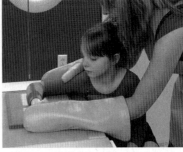

Fig. 2.62 Lateral—upper limb.

- Immobilize with clear flexible-type retention band and sandbags or with tape when necessary.
- Use the supine position with arm abducted away from body
- Include entire limb unless a specific joint or bone is indicated.
- Whether patient is supine or erect, adduct the arm and turn the forearm and wrist into a lateral position.
- Use parental assistance only if necessary; provide lead gloves and apron.

Central Ray: CR ⊥, centered to midlimb
SID: 40 inches (100 cm)
Collimation Field Size: Collimate on four sides to area of interest.

	cm	kVp	mA	Time	mAs	SID	Exposure Indicator
kVp Range:					50–60		
S							
M							
L							

Textbook, 11th ed, p. 643

Chapter 3

Humerus and Shoulder Girdle

Clavicle

Acromioclavicular (AC) Joints

Scapula

Important for humerus and shoulder projections: Do not attempt to rotate upper limb if fracture or dislocation is suspected without special orders by a physician.

(R) Routine, (S) Special

Humerus and Shoulder Girdle

74

AP: Humerus

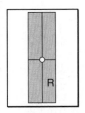

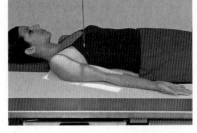

- 14 × 17 inches (35×43 cm) portrait diagonal placement if needed to include both elbow and shoulder joints.

Fig. 3.1 AP supine.

- Grid (nongrid for humerus < 4 inches [10 cm] thickness]

Position

- Patient should be erect or supine with humerus aligned to long axis of IR (unless diagonal placement is needed to **include both elbow and shoulder joints**).
- With arm abducted slightly, supinate hand for true AP (epicondyles parallel to IR).

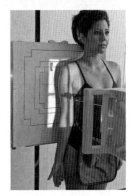

Fig. 3.2 AP erect.

Central Ray: CR ⊥, to midpoint of humerus
SID: 40 inches (100 cm)

Collimation Field Size: Collimate on sides to soft tissue borders of humerus and shoulder. (Lower margin of collimation field should include the elbow joint and approximately 1 inch [2.5 cm] minimum of proximal forearm.)

kVp Range:					80 ± 5		
	cm	kV	mA	Time	mAs	SID	Exposure Indicator
S							
M							
L							

Textbook, 11th ed, p. 185

Rotational Lateral: Humerus

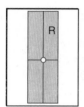

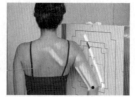

Fig. 3.3 Erect lateral (PA).

Fig. 3.4 Erect lateral (AP).

Warning: Do *not* attempt to rotate the arm if fracture or dislocation is suspected (see the following page).

- 14 × 17 inches (35 × 43 cm) portrait diagonal placement if needed to include both elbow and shoulder joints.
- Grid (nongrid for humerus < 4 inches [10 cm] thickness)

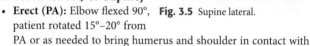

Fig. 3.5 Supine lateral.

Position (May Be Taken Erect AP or PA, or Supine)

- **Erect (PA):** Elbow flexed 90°, patient rotated 15°–20° from PA or as needed to bring humerus and shoulder in contact with IR holder (epicondyles ⊥ to IR for true lateral)
- **Erect or supine AP:** Elbow slightly flexed, arm and wrist rotated for lateral position (palm back), epicondyles ⊥ to IR
- IR centered to **include both elbow and shoulder joints**. Shield radiosensitive tissues outside region of interest.

Central Ray: CR ⊥, to midpoint of humerus

SID: 40 inches (100 cm)

Collimation Field Size: Collimate on sides to soft tissue border of humerus, ensuring that shoulder and elbow joints are included. Follow local regulations, department policy, and protocol in the use of shielding.

kVp Range:					80 ± 5		
	cm	kV	mA	Time	mAs	SID	Exposure Indicator
S							
M							
L							

Textbook, 11th ed, p. 186

Lateral: Humerus (Trauma)
Mid-to-Distal Humerus

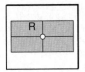

For proximal humerus, see Transthoracic Lateral or Scapular Y.

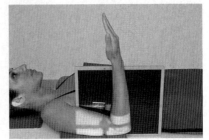

Fig. 3.6 Horizontal beam lateral cross-table, midhumerus and distal humerus.

- 14 × 17 inches (35 × 43 cm) landscape
- Grid (nongrid for humerus < 4 inches [10 cm] thickness)

Position
- With patient recumbent, perform image as a horizontal beam lateral, placing support under the arm.
- Gently lift arm, and place support block under arm; rotate hand into lateral position, if possible, for true lateral elbow projection.
- Place IR vertically between arm and thorax with top of IR at axilla (place shield between IR and patient).

Central Ray: CR horizontal and ⊥ to IR, centered to distal one-third of humerus

SID: 40 inches (100 cm)

Collimation Field Size: Collimate to soft tissue margins. Include distal and midhumerus, elbow joint, and proximal forearm.

kVp Range:						80 ± 5	
	cm	kV	mA	Time	mAs	SID	Exposure Indicator
S							
M							
L							

Textbook, 11th ed, p. 187

AP and Lateral: Humerus

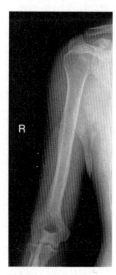

Fig. 3.7 AP humerus.

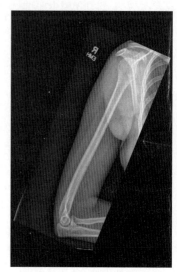

Fig. 3.8 Lateral erect humerus.

Evaluation Criteria

Anatomy Demonstrated

- AP and lateral view of the entire humerus, including elbow and glenohumeral joints

Position

- AP
- No rotation, medial and lateral epicondyles seen in profile, greater tubercle in profile laterally
- Humeral head and glenoid cavity demonstrated
- Lateral (PA)
- True lateral, epicondyles are superimposed

Exposure

- Optimal image receptor exposure and contrast; no motion
- Sharp cortical margins and clear, sharp bony trabeculation clearly demonstrated

Transthoracic Lateral: Humerus (Trauma)

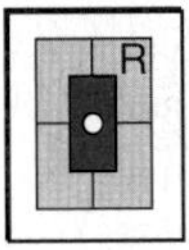

- 14 × 17 inches (35 × 43 cm) portrait
- Grid

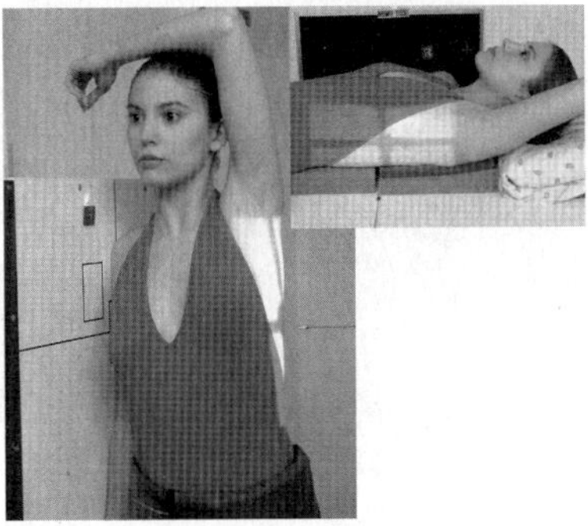

Position

- Patient should be erect (preferred) or supine.

Fig. 3.9 Transthoracic lateral.

- Affected limb should be closest to IR in neutral rotation; drop shoulder if possible.
- Raise opposite arm and place hand over top of head; elevate shoulder as much as possible to prevent superimposition of affected shoulder.
- Center mid-diaphysis of affected humerus and center of IR to CR as projected through thorax.
- Ensure the thorax is in a true lateral position or has slight anterior rotation of unaffected shoulder to minimize superimposition of humerus by thoracic vertebrae.

Central Ray: CR ⊥ to IR through thorax to midshaft of affected humerus

SID: 40 inches (100 cm)

Collimation Field Size: Collimate to soft tissue margins—entire humerus.

Respiration: Orthostatic (breathing) technique is recommended.

If Orthostatic (Breathing) Lateral Technique Performed: Minimum of 2 seconds exposure time (between 3 and 5 seconds is desirable)

	cm	kV	mA	Time	mAs	SID	Exposure Indicator
kVp Range:					85 ± 5		
S							
M							
L							

Textbook, 11th ed, p. 188

3

Humerus and Shoulder Girdle

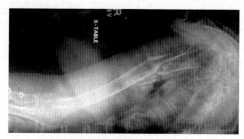

Fig. 3.10 Recumbent transthoracic lateral.

Evaluation Criteria
Anatomy Demonstrated: Lateral view of entire humerus and glenohumeral joint should be visualized through the thorax without superimposition of the opposite humerus.

Position
- Outline of the shaft of the humerus should be clearly visualized anterior to the thoracic vertebrae.
- Humeral head and glenoid cavity should be demonstrated.

Exposure
- Optimal image receptor exposure and contrast
- Overlying ribs and lung markings blurred (with orthostatic breathing technique)

AP: Shoulder
External and Internal Rotation

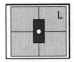

Warning: Do not attempt to rotate the arm if fracture or dislocation is suspected.

- 10 × 12 inches (24 × 30 cm) landscape (or portrait to demonstrate proximal aspect of clavicle)
- Grid

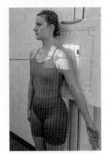

Fig. 3.11 External rotation (AP proximal humerus).

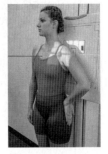

Fig. 3.12 Internal rotation (lateral proximal humerus).

Position

- Erect (seated or standing) or supine, arm slightly abducted
- Rotate body slightly toward affected side is necessary to place shoulder in contact with IR or tabletop.
- Center of IR to scapulohumeral joint and CR

External Rotation: Abduct extended arm slightly; externally rotate arm (supinate hand) until epicondyles of distal humerus are parallel to IR.

Internal Rotation: Abduct extended arm slightly; internally rotate arm (pronate hand) until epicondyles of distal humerus are perpendicular to IR.

Central Ray: CR ⊥, directed to 1 inch (2.5 cm) inferior to coracoid process

SID: 40 inches (100 cm)

Collimation Field Size: Collimate closely on four sides with lateral and upper borders adjusted to soft tissue margins.

Respiration: Suspend during exposure.

kVp Range:					80 ± 5		
	cm	kV	mA	Time	mAs	SID	Exposure Indicator
S							
M							
L							

Textbook, 11th ed, pp. 189 and 190

AP: Shoulder
External and Internal Rotation

Evaluation Criteria

Anatomy Demonstrated

- Proximal humerus and lateral two-thirds of the clavicle and upper scapula, including relationship of the humeral head to the glenoid cavity

Position:

External Rotation

- Greater tubercle visualized in full profile laterally
- Lesser tubercle superimposed over humeral head

Internal Rotation

- Lesser tubercle visualized in full profile medially
- Greater tubercle superimposed over humeral head

Exposure

- Optimal image receptor exposure and contrast; no motion
- Soft tissue detail and clear, sharp bony trabeculation clearly demonstrated

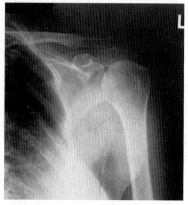

Fig. 3.13 External rotation—AP.

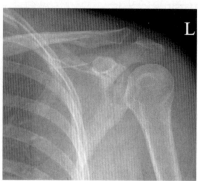

Fig. 3.14 Internal rotation—lateral.

Inferosuperior Axial (Transaxillary): Shoulder
Lawrence Method

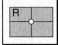

Warning: Do not attempt to rotate the arm or force abduction if fracture or dislocation is suspected.

- 8 × 10 inches (18 × 24 cm) landscape
- Grid (nongrid for shoulder < 4 inches [10 cm])

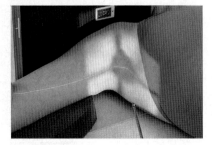

Fig. 3.15 Inferosuperior axial (Lawrence method).

Position

- Position patient supine with shoulder raised approximately 2 inches (5 cm) from tabletop by placing support under arm and shoulder to center anatomy to IR, head turned away from IR.
- Arm should be abducted 90° from body, if possible.
- Rotate arm externally, with hand supinated.

Note: An **alternative position** is exaggerated **external** rotation with the thumb pointed down and posteriorly approximately 45°. Recommended to rule out a Hills-Sachs defect.

Central Ray: CR horizontal, directed 25°–30° medially to axilla and humeral head, less angle if arm is not abducted 90° (place tube next to table or stretcher at same level as axilla)

SID: 40 inches (100 cm)

Collimation Field Size: Collimate closely on four sides.

Respiration: Suspend during exposure.

kVp Range:					80 ± 5		
	cm	kV	mA	Time	mAs	SID	Exposure Indicator
S							
M							
L							

Textbook, 11th ed, p. 191

3

Humerus and Shoulder Girdle

Inferosuperior Axial (transaxillary): Shoulder
Lawrence Method

Evaluation Criteria
Anatomy Demonstrated

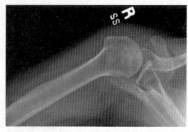

- Lateral view of proximal humerus in relationship to the scapulohumeral cavity
- Coracoid process of scapula and lesser tubercle of humerus are seen in profile.
- The spine of the scapula is seen on edge below the scapulohumeral joint.

Fig. 3.16 Inferosuperior axial (Lawrence method).

Position
- Affected arm abducted approximately 90° from the body.

Exposure
- Optimal image receptor exposure and contrast; no motion
- Soft tissue detail and clear, sharp bony trabeculation clearly demonstrated

PA Axial Transaxillary: Shoulder (Nontrauma)
Bernageau Method

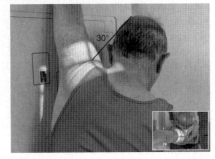

Fig. 3.17 PA transaxillary (Bernageau method).

Warning: Do *not* attempt to rotate, force extension, or abduct the arm if a fracture or dislocation is suspected.

- 8 × 10 inches (18 × 24 cm) or 10 × 12 inches (24 × 30 cm) portrait
- Grid (nongrid for shoulder < 4 inches [10 cm])

Position

- Patient recumbent or erect PA
- The patient is positioned 60°–70° from PA, rotating toward the affected side. Affected arm is raised superiorly to 160° to 180° flexion.
- Head is turned away from affected arm.

Central Ray: CR is directed 30° caudally and centered at the level of the scapular spine to pass through the scapulohumeral joint.

SID: 40 inches (100 cm)

Collimation Field Size: Collimate closely on four sides.

Respiration: Suspend during exposure.

kVp Range:					80 ± 5	
	cm	kV	mA	Time	mAs	SID	Exposure Indicator
S							
M							
L							

Textbook, 11th ed, p. 193

3

Humerus and Shoulder Girdle

PA Axial Transaxillary: Shoulder (Nontrauma)
Bernageau Method

Evaluation Criteria
Anatomy Demonstrated
- Lateral view of proximal humerus in relationship to scapulohumeral (glenohumeral) joint
- May demonstrate Bankart lesions of glenoid fossa

Position
- Coracoid process of scapula is seen on end.
- Affected arm is elevated completely.

Exposure
- Optimal image receptor exposure and contrast; no motion
- Soft tissue and clear, sharp bony trabeculation clearly demonstrated
- Bony margins of the acromion and coracoid process are visible through the humeral head.

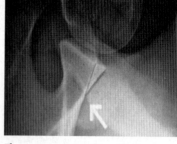

Fig. 3.18 PA transaxillary (Bernageau method). (From Pansard E, Klouche S, Billot N, et al. Reliability and validity assessment of a glenoid bone loss measurement using the Bernageau profile view in chronic anterior shoulder instability. *J Shoulder Elbow Surg* 22(9):1193–1198, 2013.)

Inferosuperior Axial: Shoulder (Nontrauma)
Clements Modification

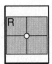

Warning: Do *not* attempt to rotate the arm or force abduction if a fracture or dislocation is suspected.

- 8 × 10 inches (18 × 24 cm) portrait
- Nongrid

Position

- Patient in lateral recumbent position; lying on unaffected side
- Affected arm up
- Abduct arm 90° from body, if possible

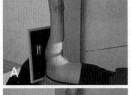

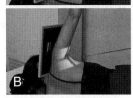

Fig. 3.19 Inferosuperior axial (Clements modification).

Central Ray: Direct horizontal CR perpendicular to the IR (angle the tube 5°–15° toward the axilla if the patient cannot abduct the arm 90°)

SID: 40 inches (100 cm)

Collimation Field Size: Collimate closely on four sides.

Respiration: Suspend during exposure.

	cm	kV	mA	Time	mAs	SID	Exposure Indicator
S							
M							
L							

kVp Range: 80 ± 5

Textbook, 11th ed, p. 192

Inferosuperior Axial: Shoulder
Clements Modification

Evaluation Criteria

Anatomy Demonstrated

- Lateral view of proximal humerus in relationship to the scapulohumeral joint

Position

- Arm is abducted 90° from the body.

Exposure

- Optimal image receptor exposure and contrast; no motion
- Soft tissue and clear, sharp bony trabeculation clearly demonstrated
- Bony margins of the acromion and distal clavicle are visible through the humeral head.

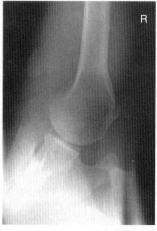

Fig. 3.20 Inferosuperior axial (Clements modification). (From Frank ED, Long BW, Smith BJ: *Merrill's atlas of radiographic positioning and procedures*, ed 11, St. Louis, 2007, Mosby.)

Superoinferior Transaxillary Projection

Warning: Do *not* attempt to rotate the arm or force abduction if a fracture or dislocation is suspected.

- 8 × 10 inches (18 × 24 cm) or 10 x 12 inches (24 x 30 cm) landscape
- Nongrid

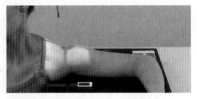

Fig. 3.21 Superoinferior Transaxillary

Position

- Elbow is flexed to 90°
- Patient leans laterally over the IR, abducting their humerus much as possible
- Tilt the patient's head away from the affected shoulder

Central Ray

- CR is directed perpendicular to the glenoid fossa, which is perpendicular to the line between the AC joint and the superior angle of the scapula, approximately 5-15° laterally (toward elbow)

SID: 40 inches (100 cm)

Collimation Field Size: Collimate closely on four sides.

Respiration: Suspend during exposure.

kVp Range:					75 ± 5	
	cm	kV	mA	Time	mAs	SID	Exposure Indicator
S							
M							
L							

Textbook, 11th ed, p. 194

Superoinferior Transaxillary Projection

Evaluation Criteria

Anatomy Demonstrated

- Lateral view of proximal humerus in relationship to scapulohumeral (glenohumeral) articulation is visualized.

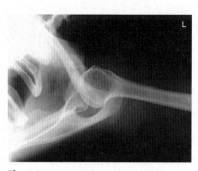

Fig. 3.22 Superoinferior Transaxillary. (From Rollins J, Long B, Curtis C: *Merrill's atlas of radiographic positioning and procedures*, ed 15, St. Louis, 2023, Elsevier).

Position

- Arm is abducted from the body

Exposure

- Optimal image receptor exposure and contrast with **no motion** demonstrate clear, sharp bony trabecular markings and pertinent soft tissue anatomy.
- Bony margins of the acromion and coracoid process are visible through the humeral head

AP Oblique–Glenoid Cavity: Shoulder
Grashey Method

This is a special
projection for visu-
alizing glenoid cav-
ity in profile with
open joint space.

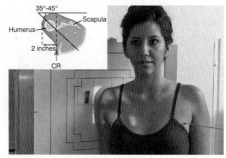

Fig. 3.23 AP oblique—Grashey method.

- 8 × 10 inches
  (18 × 24 cm) or
  10 × 12 inches
  (24 × 30 cm) landscape
- Grid

Position

- Patient should be erect (preferred) or supine.
- Rotate body 35°–45° toward affected side (body of scapula should be parallel with IR), hand and arm in neutral rotation.
- Center midscapulohumeral joint and IR to CR; 2 inches (5 cm) above shoulder and side of IR is approximately 2 inches (5 cm) from lateral border of humerus.
- Abduct arm slightly with arm flexed and in neutral rotation.

Central Ray

- CR ⊥, to scapulohumeral joint, approximately 2 inches (5 cm) inferior and 2 inches (5 cm) medial from the superolateral border of shoulder

SID: 40 inches (100 cm)

Collimation Field Size: Collimate so upper and lateral borders of the field are to the soft tissue margins.

Respiration: Suspend during exposure.

	cm	kV	mA	Time	mAs	SID	Exposure Indicator
kVp Range:					80 ± 5		
S							
M							
L							

Textbook, 11th ed, p. 195

AP Oblique: Shoulder
Grashey Method

Evaluation Criteria

Anatomy Demonstrated

- Glenoid cavity should be seen in profile without superimposition of humeral head.

Position

- Scapulohumeral joint space is open.
- Anterior and posterior rims of glenoid cavity are superimposed.

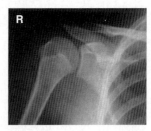

Fig. 3.24 AP oblique—Grashey method.

Exposure

- Optimal image receptor exposure and contrast; no motion
- Soft tissue margins and clear, sharp bony trabeculation clearly demonstrated

Tangential–Intertubercular (Bicipital) Sulcus: Shoulder
Fisk Modification

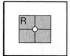

- 8 × 10 inches (18 × 24 cm) or 10 × 12 inches (24 × 30 cm), landscape
- Nongrid

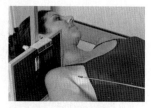

Fig. 3.25 Supine inferosuperior tangential projection (CR 15°–20° from horizontal).

Position

- Supine or erect. Palpate anterior humeral head to locate groove.

Seated: (Fisk Modification): Patient standing, leaning over the end of the table to place humerus 10°–15° from vertical, CR vertical, ⊥ to IR; hand supinated holding IR, head turned away from affected side (lead shield placed between back of IR and forearm)

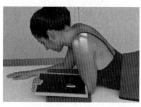

Fig. 3.26 Erect superoinferior tangential (humerus 15°–20° from vertical, CR, ⊥ to IR).

Supine

- Abduct arm slightly, supinate hand
- Vertical IR placed on table against top of shoulder and against neck (head turned away from affected side)
- CR 10°–15° posterior from horizontal, directed to groove at midanterior margin of humeral head

SID: 40 inches (100 cm)

Collimation Field Size: Collimate closely on four sides to area of anterior humeral head.

Respiration: Suspend during exposure.

	cm	kV	mA	Time	mAs	SID	Exposure Indicator
S							
M							
L							

kVp Range: 75 ± 5

Tangential–Intertubercular (Bicipital) Sulcus: Shoulder
Fisk Modification

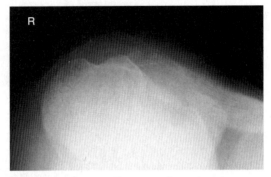

Fig. 3.27 Erect tangential projection (intertubercular groove).

Evaluation Criteria
Anatomy Demonstrated
- Humeral tubercles and intertubercular groove seen in profile

Position
- Intertubercular groove and tubercles in profile
- No superimposition of acromion process

Exposure
- Optimal image receptor exposure and contrast; no motion
- Sharp borders and clear, sharp bony trabeculation clearly demonstrating intertubercular sulcus seen through soft tissue

PA Oblique: Shoulder (Trauma)
Scapular Y Lateral and Neer Method

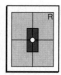

Warning: Do *not* attempt to rotate the arm if a fracture or dislocation is suspected.

- 10 × 12 inches (24 × 30 cm) portrait
- Grid

Position

- Patient should be erect (preferred) or recumbent.
- Patient PA, then rotate affected shoulder into a 45°–60° posterior oblique as for a lateral scapula (body of scapula perpendicular to IR).

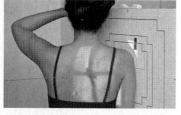

Fig. 3.28 PA oblique (scapular Y lateral) with CR ⊥.

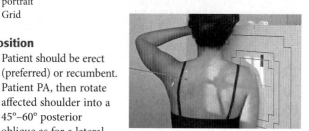

Fig. 3.29 Tangential (Neer method) with CR 10°–15° caudad.

- Unaffected arm should be up in front of patient, affected arm down (**do not move with possible fracture or dislocation**).
- Center scapulohumeral joint and CR.

Central Ray: CR ⊥ to scapulohumeral joint

Neer Method: Angle CR 10°–15° caudad to better demonstrate the acromiohumeral space (supraspinatus outlet), CR to superior margin of humeral head

SID: 40 inches (100 cm)

Collimation Field Size: Collimate on four sides to area of interest.

Respiration: Suspend during exposure.

kVp Range:					80 ± 5		
	cm	kV	mA	Time	mAs	SID	Exposure Indicator
S							
M							
L							

Textbook, 11th ed, pp. 200 and 201

PA Oblique: Shoulder (Trauma)
Scapular Y Lateral and Neer Method

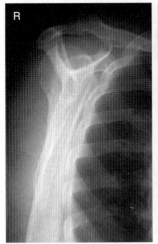

Fig. 3.30 PA oblique (scapular Y lateral) with no dislocation.

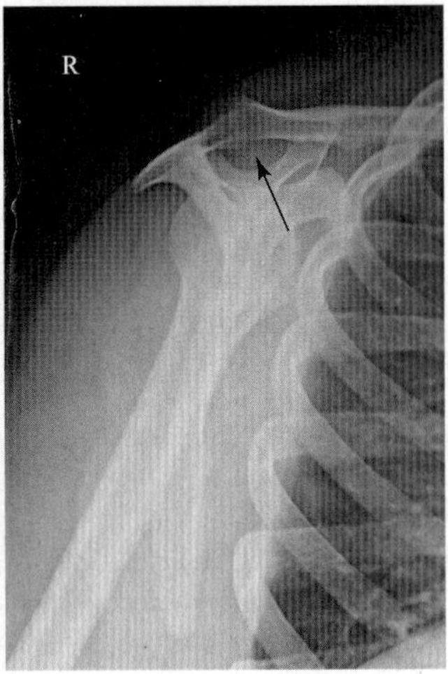

Fig. 3.31 Tangential projection (Neer method).

Evaluation Criteria

Anatomy Demonstrated

- **Scapular Y:** True lateral view of the scapula, proximal humerus, and scapulohumeral joint
- **Neer method:** Supraspinatus outlet region is open.

Position

- **Scapular Y:** The acromion and coracoid processes should appear as nearly symmetric upper limbs of the "Y."
  - The humeral head should appear superimposed over the base of the "Y" if the humerus is not dislocated.
  - Thin body of the scapula is seen on end without rib superimposition. Upper limb is not elevated or moved with possible fracture or dislocation
- **Neer method:** Thin body of the scapula is seen on end; humeral head below supraspinatus outlet *(arrow)*.

Exposure

- Optimal image receptor exposure and contrast; no motion. Visualize sharp bony borders and the outline of the body of the scapula through the proximal humerus.

AP–Neutral Rotation: Shoulder (Trauma)

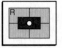

Warning: Do *not* attempt to rotate the arm if a fracture or dislocation is suspected; perform in neutral rotation, which generally places the humerus in an oblique position.

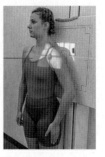

Fig. 3.32 AP—neutral rotation.

- 10 × 12 inches (24 × 30 cm) landscape (or portrait to show more of humerus if injury includes proximal half of humerus)
- Grid

Position

- Patient should be erect (seated or standing) or supine, arm slightly abducted.
- Rotate body slightly toward affected side if necessary to place shoulder in contact with IR or tabletop.
- Position patient to center scapulohumeral joint to IR.
- Place patient's arm at side in "as is" neutral rotation. (Epicondyles generally are approximately 45° to plane of IR.)

Central Ray: CR ⊥, directed to **midscapulohumeral joint**, which is approximately ¾ inch (2 cm) inferior and slightly lateral to coracoid process

SID: 40 inches (100 cm)

Collimation Field Size: Collimate on four sides to area of interest, with lateral and upper borders adjusted to soft tissue margins.

Respiration: Suspend during exposure.

	cm	kV	mA	Time	mAs	SID	Exposure Indicator
kVp Range:					80 ± 5		
S							
M							
L							

Textbook, 11th ed, p. 198

Transthoracic Lateral: Shoulder (Trauma)
Lawrence Method

- 10 × 12 inches (24 × 30 cm) portrait
- Grid
- Orthostatic (breathing) technique is preferred if patient can cooperate.

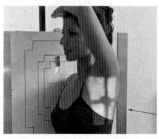

Fig. 3.33 Erect transthoracic lateral.

Position

- Patient should be erect (preferred) or supine, affected arm against IR, arm at side in neutral position.
- Place patient in lateral position with side of interest against IR.
- Raise unaffected arm above head **or** angle CR 10°–15° cephalad to prevent superimposition of unaffected shoulder.

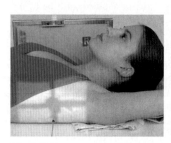

Fig. 3.34 Supine transthoracic lateral.

- Ensure that thorax is in a true lateral position, or slight anterior rotation of unaffected shoulder.

Central Ray: CR ⊥, through thorax to level of affected surgical neck
SID: 40 inches (100 cm)
Collimation Field Size: Collimate on four sides to area of interest.
Respiration: Expose on full inspiration; orthostatic (breathing) technique preferred.

kVp Range:						85 ± 5	
	cm	kV	mA	Time	mAs	SID	Exposure Indicator
S							
M							
L							

Textbook, 11th ed, p. 202

Transthoracic Lateral: Shoulder (Trauma)
Lawrence Method

Evaluation Criteria

Anatomy Demonstrated

- Lateral view of proximal humerus and scapulohumeral joint should be visualized.

Position

- Shaft of the proximal humerus should be clearly visualized.
- Humeral head and the glenoid cavity should be visualized.

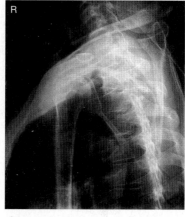

Fig. 3.35 Erect transthoracic lateral.

Exposure

- Optimal image receptor exposure and contrast; no motion of humerus during exposure
- Ribs and lungs should be blurred due to breathing technique, but bony outlines of the humerus should appear sharp.

Humerus and Shoulder Girdle

AP Apical Oblique Axial: Shoulder (Trauma)
Garth Method

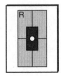

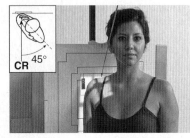

Optional projection for acute shoulder trauma, demonstrating shoulder dislocations, glenoid fractures, and Hill-Sachs lesions

Fig. 3.36 Erect apical oblique (45° posterior oblique, CR 45° caudad).

- 10 × 12 inches (24 × 30 cm) portrait
- Grid

Position

- Erect (preferred) or recumbent (if necessary)
- Rotate body 45° toward affected side (posterior surface of affected shoulder against IR).
- Adjust IR so that 45° CR projects scapulohumeral joint to the center of IR.
- Flex affected elbow and place across chest, or, with trauma, place arm at side as is.

Central Ray: CR 45° caudad, centered to scapulohumeral joint.

Hint: CR enters just inferior to coracoid process.

SID: 40 inches (100 cm)

Collimation Field Size: Collimate on four sides to area of interest.

Respiration: Suspend during exposure.

	cm	kV	mA	Time	mAs	SID	Exposure Indicator
S							
M							
L							

kVp Range: 80 ± 5

Textbook, 11th ed, p. 202

AP Apical Oblique Axial: Shoulder (Trauma)
Garth Method

Evaluation Criteria

Anatomy Demonstrated
- Humeral head, glenoid cavity, and neck and head of scapula free of superimposition

Position
- The coracoid process is projected over part of the humeral head, which appears elongated.
- Acromion and AC joint are projected superior to the humeral head.

Exposure
- Optimal image receptor exposure and contrast; no motion
- Soft tissue detail and clear, sharp bony trabeculation clearly demonstrated; no motion

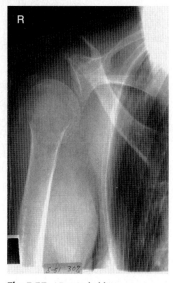

Fig. 3.37 AP apical oblique.

Apical AP Axial: Shoulder

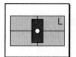

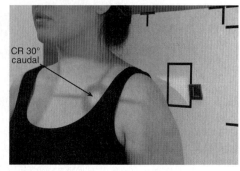

Fig. 3.38 Erect apical AP axial (CR 30° caudad).

Demonstrates narrowing of acromiohumeral space and possible spurring of the anteroinferior aspect of acromion.

- 8 × 10 inches (18 × 24 cm) or10 × 12 inches (24 × 30 cm) landscape
- Grid

Position
- Patient should be erect (preferred) or supine.
- Center midscapulohumeral joint to CR and to center of IR.
- Adjust IR so that top of IR is approximately 1 inch (2.5 cm) above shoulder and side of IR is approximately 2 inches (5 cm) from lateral border of humerus.

Central Ray: Angle CR 30° caudad entering ½ inch (1.25 cm) above **coracoid process**

SID: 40 inches (100 cm)

Collimation Field Size: Collimate to soft tissue margins of shoulder

Respiration: Expose upon suspended respiration

kVp Range:					80 ± 5		
	cm	kV	mA	Time	mAs	SID	Exposure Indicator
S							
M							
L							

Textbook, 11th ed, p. 196

Apical AP Axial: Shoulder

Evaluation Criteria

Anatomy Demonstrated

- The anteroinferior aspect of the acromion process and acromiohumeral joint space is open.
- Proximal humerus is projected in neutral rotation position.

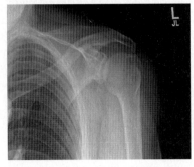

Fig. 3.39 Apical AP axial.

Position

- Acromiohumeral space is more open as compared to routine AP shoulder projection.
- Anteroinferior aspect of acromion is demonstrated.

Exposure

- Optimal image receptor exposure and contrast; no motion
- Soft tissue detail and clear, sharp bony trabeculation clearly demonstrated

AP and AP Axial: Clavicle

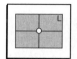

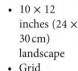

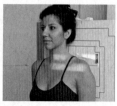

Fig. 3.40 AP, 0°.

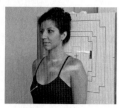

Fig. 3.41 AP axial, 15° to 30° cephalad.

- 10 × 12 inches (24 × 30 cm) landscape
- Grid

Position

- Patient erect (preferred) or recumbent. Posterior shoulder should be in contact with IR or tabletop, without rotation of body.
- Center clavicle and IR to CR (midway between jugular notch medially and lateral portion at AC joint above shoulder)

Central Ray: CR to midclavicle

AP: CR ⊥, to midclavicle

AP Axial: Angled 15°–30° cephalad to midclavicle* (thin shoulders require 5°–15° more angle than thick shoulders)

Note: Departmental routines may include AP 0°, or axial AP, or both.

SID: 40 inches (100 cm)

Collimation Field Size: Collimate to area of clavicle. (Ensure that both AC and sternoclavicular joints are included.)

Respiration: Suspend respiration at end of inhalation.

* AP lordotic position can be performed rather than angling CR for AP axial.

kVp Range:							80 ± 5
	cm	kV	mA	Time	mAs	SID	Exposure Indicator
S							
M							
L							

Textbook, 11th ed, p. 203

AP and AP Axial: Clavicle

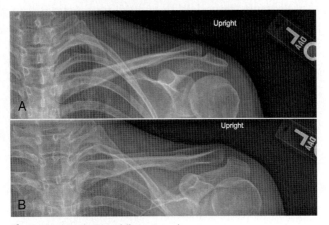

Fig. 3.42 AP and AP axial (lower image).

Evaluation Criteria

Anatomy Demonstrated

- **AP 0°:** Entire clavicle including both AC and SC joints and acromion
- **AP axial:** Entire clavicle including AC and SC joints and acromion above the scapula and ribs

Position

- **AP 0°:** Entire clavicle from AC to SC joint
- **AP axial:** Clavicle projected above scapula, second and third ribs. Only medial portion of clavicle will be superimposed by first and second ribs.

Exposure

- Optimal image receptor exposure and contrast; no motion
- Soft tissue detail and clear, sharp bony trabeculation clearly demonstrated

Humerus and Shoulder Girdle

AP (Bilateral): Acromioclavicular (AC) Joints
Pearson Method, With and Without Weights

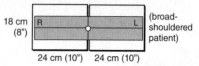

Warning: Shoulder or clavicle projections should be completed first to rule out fracture, or this image may be taken without weights first and checked before it is taken with weights.

- 14 × 17 inches (35 × 43 cm) landscape, or (2) 10 × 12 inches (24 × 30 cm) landscape for unilateral exposures
- For broad-shouldered patients, **two 8 × 10 inches (18 × 24 cm) IRs landscape**, placed side by side and exposed simultaneously to include both AC joints on a single exposure
- Grid (nongrid for shoulder < 4 inches [10 cm])
- "With weights" and "without weights" markers

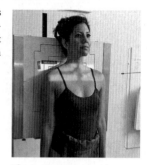

Fig. 3.43 Bilateral with weights.

Position
- Patient should be erect and standing (preferred) or seated.
- Posterior shoulders against IR with equal weight on both feet; arms at side; no rotation of shoulders or pelvis; and looking straight ahead (may be taken seated if patient's condition requires)
- **Two sets** of bilateral AC joints are taken in the same position, one **without weights** and one **stress view with weights** (8–10 lbs. [3.5–4.5 kg] minimum, 5–8 lbs. [2–3.5 kg] for smaller patients). Center midline of IR to CR (top of IR should be approximately 2 inches [5 cm] above shoulders).

Central Ray
- CR ⊥, to midpoint between AC joints, 1 inch (2.5 cm) above jugular notch
- Unilateral study: CR center 1 inch (2.5 cm) below affected AC joint

SID: 40 inches (100 cm); 72 inches (180 cm) recommended for bilateral studies with a single IR

Collimation Field Size: Long, narrow horizontal exposure field; upper light border should be to upper shoulder soft tissue margins.

Respiration: Suspend during exposure.

Alternative AP Axial Projection (Zanca Method): A 15° cephalic angle centered at the level of the affected AC joint to rule out subluxation or dislocation of AC joint

Alternative AP Axial Projection (Zanca Method): A 10° to 15° cephalic angle is centered at the level of the affected AC joint, which projects the AC joint superior to the acromion, providing optimal visualization. The Zanca method also uses 50% less kilovoltage than a standard glenohumeral exposure to allow better visualization of the soft-tissue and joint detail of the AC joint. This projection may be performed for suspected AC joint subluxation or dislocation as well as for soft-tissue pathologies. (See textbook, Chapter 5 for further information on Zanca method)

kVp Range:			80 ± 5 (grid recommended for larger shoulders)				
	cm	kV	mA	Time	mAs	SID	Exposure Indicator
S							
M							
L							

Textbook, 11th ed, p. 204

AP (Bilateral): AC Joint
Pearson Method, With and Without Weights

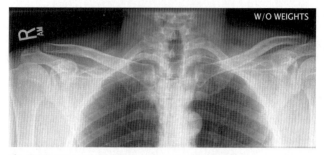

Fig. 3.44 AP acromioclavicular joints without weights.

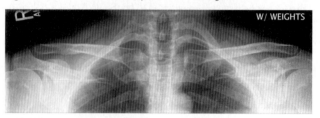

Fig. 3.45 AP acromioclavicular joints with weights.

Evaluation Criteria

Anatomy Demonstrated
- Both AC joints, entire clavicles and SC joints included

Position
- Both AC joints are on the same horizontal plane.
- No rotation, symmetric SC joints

Exposure
- Optimal image receptor exposure and contrast; no motion
- Bony margins and clear, sharp bony trabeculation clearly demonstrated

AP: Scapula

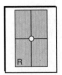

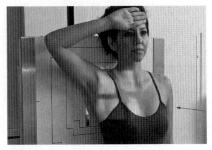

Fig. 3.46 AP scapula erect.

- 10 × 12 inches (24 × 30 cm) portrait
- Grid

Position

- Patient should be erect (preferred) or supine. Posterior surface of shoulder is in direct contact with tabletop or IR without rotation of thorax.
- Adjust IR to center to CR. Top of IR should be approximately 2 inches (5 cm) above shoulder, and lateral border of IR should be approximately 2 inches (5 cm) from lateral margin of rib cage.
- Gently abduct arm 90°, if possible; supinate hand (abduction results in less superimposition of scapula by ribs).

Central Ray: CR ⊥, to midscapula (2 inches [5 cm] inferior to coracoid process and 2 inches [5 cm] medial from lateral border of patient)

SID: 40 inches (100 cm)

Collimation Field Size: Collimate on four sides of scapula borders.

Respiration: Orthostatic (breathing) technique is preferred, or suspend respiration during exposure.

	cm	kV	mA	Time	mAs	SID	Exposure Indicator
S							
M							
L							

kVp Range: 80 ± 5

Textbook, 11th ed, p. 206

Humerus and Shoulder Girdle

3

Lateral (Erect and Recumbent): Scapula

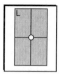

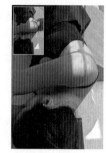

- 10 × 12 inches (24 × 30 cm) portrait

Fig. 3.47 Recumbent (Elevate affected aside away from IR).

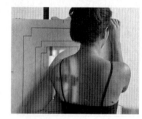

Fig. 3.48 For body of scapula.

Fig. 3.49 Superior scapula (acromion or coracoid process), place arm down, flex elbow.

Position
- Patient should be erect (preferred) or recumbent.
- Patient's face is toward IR in anterior oblique position.
- If area of interest is body of scapula, with patient's arm up, have patient reach across and grasp opposite shoulder.
- If area of interest is acromion and coracoid processes, have patient drop affected arm, flex elbow, and place arm behind lower back with arm partially abducted, or just let arm hang down at patient's side.
- Palpate borders of scapula, and rotate thorax until body of scapula is perpendicular to IR (will vary from 45°–60° rotation).

Central Ray: CR ⊥, to midvertebral border of scapula
SID: 40 inches (100 cm)
Collimation Field Size: Closely collimate to area of scapula.
Respiration: Suspend during exposure.

	cm	kV	mA	Time	mAs	SID	Exposure Indicator
kVp Range:					80 ± 5		
S							
M							
L							

Textbook, 11th ed, pp. 207 and 208.

3

Humerus and Shoulder Girdle

AP and Lateral: Scapula

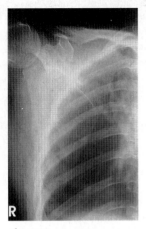

Fig. 3.50 AP scapula.

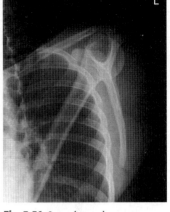

Fig. 3.51 Lateral scapula.

Evaluation Criteria

Anatomy Demonstrated
- **AP:** Entire scapula
- **Lateral:** Entire scapula in a lateral position

Position
- **AP:** Lateral border of scapula free of superimposition
- **Lateral:** Humerus not superimposing over region of interest; ribs free of superimposition by body of scapula

Exposure
- Optimal image receptor exposure and contrast; no motion
- Sharp bony borders and trabeculation clearly demonstrated

3

Humerus and Shoulder Girdle

Lower Limb

4

Lower Limb

(R) Routine, (S) Special

Digital Imaging Considerations

- **Four-sided collimation:** Collimate to the area of interest with a minimum of two (four is preferred) collimation parallel borders clearly demonstrated on the image.
- **Accurate centering:** The body part and the central ray (CR) should be centered to the IR.
- **Grid use with cassette-less systems:** Anatomy thickness and kVp range are deciding factors for whether a grid is to be used. With cassette-less systems, it may be impractical and difficult to remove the grid. Therefore, the grid is commonly left in place even for smaller body parts measuring < 4 inches (10 cm) or less. If the grid is left in place, ensure the CR is centered to the grid. Virtual grid technology may eliminate the need for a physical grid

Multiple Exposures per Imaging Plate

Placing multiple images on the same IP is not recommended. However, if doing so, careful collimation and lead masking must be used to prevent preexposure of other images.

AP: Toes

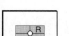

Alternative Routine: May include entire foot on AP toe projection for possible secondary trauma to other parts of foot (see AP foot).

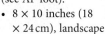

Fig. 4.1 AP second digit, CR 10°–15° toward calcaneus.

- 8 × 10 inches (18 × 24 cm), landscape
- Nongrid
- Lead masking with multiple exposures on same IR

Position

- Patient should be supine or seated on table with knee flexed, plantar surface of foot resting on IR.
- Center and align long axis of affected toe(s) to the portion of IR being exposed.

Central Ray

- CR angled 10°–15° to calcaneus (⊥ to long axis of digits)
- CR centered to MTP joint(s) of interest

SID: 40 inches (100 cm)

Collimation Field Size: Collimate on four sides to area of interest to include soft tissue margins.

	cm	kVp	mA	Time	mAs	SID	Exposure Indicator
S							
M							
L							

kVp Range: 50–60

Textbook, 11th ed, p. 228

AP Oblique: Toes

- 8 × 10 inches (18 × 24 cm), landscape
- Nongrid
- Lead masking with multiple exposures on same IR

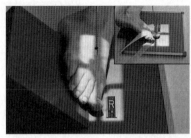

Fig. 4.2 Medial oblique rotation (first digit).

Position

- Patient supine or seated on table, with knee flexed, foot resting on IR
- Align long axis of affected toe(s) to the portion of IR being exposed.
- Oblique foot 30°–45° medially for first to

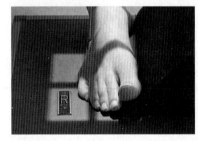

Fig. 4.3 Lateral oblique rotation (fourth digit).

third digits, and laterally for fourth and fifth digits. Place support under foot as shown.

Central Ray: CR ⊥, centered to MTP joint(s) of interest

SID: 40 inches (100 cm)

Collimation Field Size: Collimate on four sides to area of interest to include soft tissue margins.

	cm	kVp	mA	Time	mAs	SID	Exposure Indicator
S							
M							
L							

kVp Range: 50–60

Textbook, 11th ed, p. 229

AP and AP Oblique: Toes

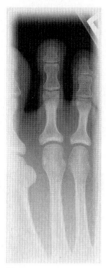

Fig. 4.4 AP toe.

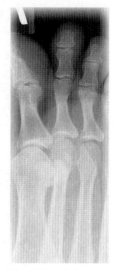

Fig. 4.5 Medial oblique toe.

Evaluation Criteria

Anatomy Demonstrated

- **AP and AP Oblique:** Entire digit and minimum of one-half of affected metatarsal

Position

- **AP:** No overlap of surrounding digits and metatarsals; no rotation, equal concavity on both sides of shafts of phalanges and metatarsals
- **AP Oblique:** Increased concavity on one side of phalangeal shaft

Exposure

- Optimal image receptor exposure and contrast; no motion
- Sharp cortical margins and bony trabeculae clearly demonstrated

Lateral: Toes

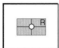

- 8 × 10 inches (18 × 24 cm), landscape
- Nongrid
- Lead masking with multiple exposures on same IR

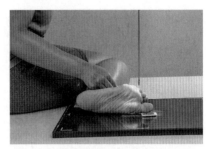

Fig. 4.6 Lateromedial (first digit).

Position

- Patient should be seated or recumbent on tabletop.
- Carefully use tape or radiolucent gauze to isolate unaffected digits as shown.
- Rotate affected leg and foot medially (lateromedial) for

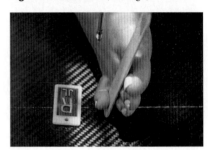

Fig. 4.7 Mediolateral (fourth digit).

first, second, and third digits (first digit down) and laterally (mediolateral) for fourth and fifth digits (first digit up).

Central Ray: CR ⊥ to IP joint for first digit, and to PIP joint for second to fifth digits

SID: 40 inches (100 cm)

Collimation Field Size: Collimate closely to digit of interest to include soft tissue margins.

	cm	kVp	mA	Time	mAs	SID	Exposure Indicator
kVp Range:					50–60		
S							
M							
L							

Textbook, 11th ed, p. 230

Lower Limb

4

Tangential: Toes–Sesamoids

- 8 × 10 inches (18 × 24 cm), landscape

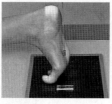

Fig. 4.8 Patient prone.

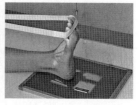

Fig. 4.9 Alternative supine position.

- Nongrid
- Lead masking with multiple exposures on same IR

Position
- Patient prone with foot and great toe carefully dorsiflexed so the plantar surface forms a 15°–20° angle from vertical, if possible (adjust CR angle, as needed)

Alternative Supine Position: May be a more tolerable position for patients to maintain if in great pain. Long strip of gauze is needed for the patient to hold the toes as shown.

Central Ray: CR ⊥, or angled, as needed, depending on amount of dorsiflexion of foot, centered to head of first metatarsal

SID: 40 inches (100 cm)

Collimation Field Size: Collimate closely to area of interest; include distal first, second, and third metatarsals for possible sesamoids.

	cm	kVp	mA	Time	mAs	SID	Exposure Indicator
S							
M							
L							

kVp Range: 50–60

Textbook, 11th ed, p. 231

4

Lower Limb

Lateral: Toes

Evaluation Criteria
Anatomy Demonstrated
- Entire digit, including proximal phalanx

Position
- True lateral of digit demonstrates increased concavity on anterior surface of the distal phalanx and posterior surface of the proximal phalanx.
- No superimposition of adjoining digits
- Proximal phalanx visualized through superimposed structures

Exposure
- Optimal image receptor exposure and contrast sufficient to visualize soft tissue and bony portions; no motion

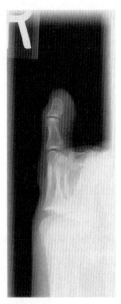

Fig. 4.10 Lateromedial second digit.

Tangential: Sesamoids

Evaluation Criteria
Anatomy Demonstrated
- Sesamoid bones in profile

Position
- No superimposition of sesamoids and first to third distal metatarsals in profile

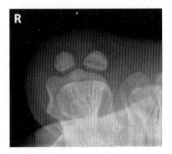

Fig. 4.11 Tangential sesamoids.

Exposure
- Optimal image receptor exposure and contrast; no motion
- Soft tissue, trabeculae, and sharp cortical margins clearly demonstrated

Dorsoplantar AP: Foot

- 10 × 12 inches (24 × 30 cm), portrait
- Nongrid
- Lead masking with multiple exposures on same IR

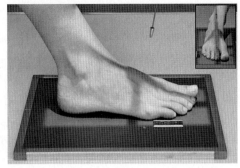

Fig. 4.12 AP foot, CR 10° posteriorly.

Position

- Patient should be supine or seated with plantar surface flat on IR, aligned lengthwise to the portion of IR being exposed.
- Flex knee and place plantar surface (sole) of affected foot flat on IR.
- Extend (plantar flex) foot, but maintain plantar surface resting flat and firmly on IR.

Central Ray: CR ⊥ to metatarsals, which is about 10° posteriorly (toward heel), centered to base of third metatarsal

SID: 40 inches (100 cm)

Collimation Field Size: Collimate on four sides to area of interest to include soft tissue margins.

	cm	kVp	mA	Time	mAs	SID	Exposure Indicator
kVp Range:					55–65		
S							
M							
L							

Textbook, 11th ed, p. 232

AP Medial Oblique: Foot

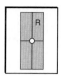

- 10 × 12 inches (24 × 30 cm), portrait
- Nongrid
- Lead masking with multiple exposures on same IR

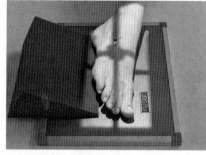

Fig. 4.13 30°–40° medial oblique.

Position

- Patient should be supine or seated with foot centered lengthwise to the portion of IR being exposed.
- Oblique foot 30°–40° medially, and support with 45° radiolucent angle block and sandbags to prevent slippage.
- **Note 1:** A higher arch requires nearer 40° oblique and a low arch "flat foot" nearer 30°.
- **Note 2:** A 30° lateral oblique projection will demonstrate the space between first and second metatarsals and between first and second cuneiforms.

Central Ray: CR ⊥, centered to base of third metatarsal

SID: 40 inches (100 cm)

Collimation Field Size: Collimate on four sides to area of interest to include soft tissue margins.

	cm	kVp	mA	Time	mAs	SID	Exposure Indicator
S							
M							
L							

kVp Range: 60–70

Textbook, 11th ed, p. 233

AP and AP Medial Oblique: Foot

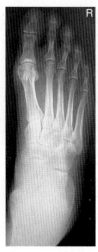

Fig. 4.14 AP foot.

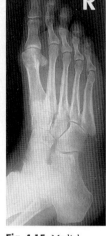

Fig. 4.15 Medial oblique foot.

Evaluation Criteria

Anatomy Demonstrated
- **AP and AP medial oblique:** Entire foot, including tarsals, metatarsals, and phalanges

Position:
AP
- No rotation with tarsals superimposed

AP Medial Oblique
- Third to fifth metatarsals free of superimposition
- Cuboid clearly demonstrated; base of fifth metatarsal seen in profile

Exposure
- Optimal image receptor exposure and contrast; no motion
- Soft tissue and sharp bony trabeculation clearly demonstrated

Mediolateral or Lateromedial: Foot

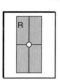

- 8 × 10 inches (18 × 24 cm), portrait

or

- 10 × 12 inches (24 × 30 cm), portrait for large foot
- Nongrid

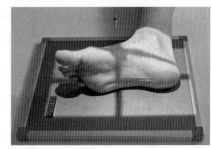

Fig. 4.16 Mediolateral foot.

Position (Mediolateral)

- Patient should be recumbent, on affected side, knee flexed about 45° with unaffected leg behind patient to prevent over-rotation.

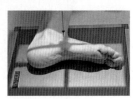

Fig. 4.17 Lateromedial foot.

- Carefully dorsiflex foot if possible, to assist in positioning for a true lateral foot and ankle.
- Place support under affected knee and leg, as needed, to place plantar surface of foot perpendicular to IR.

Lateromedial Projection: May be easier to achieve a true lateral if patient's condition allows this position.

Central Ray: CR ⊥, centered to area of base of third metatarsal

SID: 40 inches (100 cm)

Collimation Field Size: Collimate on four sides to area of interest to include soft tissue margins.

	cm	kVp	mA	Time	mAs	SID	Exposure Indicator
kVp Range:					60–70		
S							
M							
L							

Textbook, 11th ed, p. 234

4

Lower Limb

Lateral-Mediolateral or Lateromedial: Foot

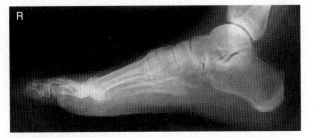

Fig. 4.18 Mediolateral foot.

Evaluation Criteria

Anatomy Demonstrated
- Entire foot with ≈1 inch (2.5 cm) of distal tibia-fibula

Position
- True lateral with tibiotalar joint open
- Distal fibula superimposed by the posterior tibia, and distal metatarsals superimposed

Exposure
- Optimal image receptor exposure and contrast; no motion
- Soft tissue and sharp bony trabeculation clearly demonstrated

Weight-Bearing AP and Lateral: Foot

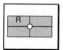

Lateral projection is most common for longitudinal arch (flat feet); AP demonstrates alignment of metatarsals and phalanges. Bilateral projections of both feet are often obtained for comparison:

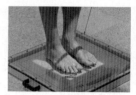

Fig. 4.19 AP-bilateral feet CR 15° posteriorly.

- 10 × 12 inches (24 × 30 cm), landscape; 14 × 17 inches (35 × 43 cm), landscape for bilateral study
- Nongrid

Position

- **AP:** Patient erect, weight evenly distributed on both feet, on one IR
- **Lateral:** Patient erect, full weight on both feet, vertical IR between feet, standing on blocks, high enough from floor for horizontal CR (R and L feet obtained for comparison)

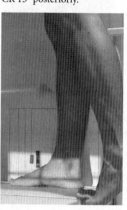

Fig. 4.20 Lateral—right foot.

Central Ray

- **AP:** CR 15° posteriorly, CR to level of base of third metatarsal, midway between feet
- **Lateral:** CR horizontal, to base of third metatarsal

SID: 40 inches (100 cm)

Collimation Field Size: Collimate on four sides to area of interest to include soft tissue margins.

kVp Range:					60–70	
	cm	kVp	mA	Time	mAs	SID	Exposure Indicator
S							
M							
L							

Textbook, 11th ed, pp. 235 and 236

Weight-Bearing AP and Lateral: Foot

Evaluation Criteria

Anatomy Demonstrated
- **AP:** Bilateral feet with soft tissue detail, including distal talus
- **Lateral:** Entire foot with 1 inch (2.5 cm) of distal tibia-fibula

Position
- **AP:** Open tarsometatarsal joints; with approximately equal spacing of second to fourth metatarsals

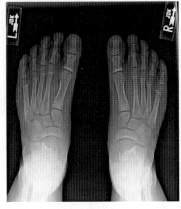

Fig. 4.21 AP weight-bearing bilateral feet.

Lateral: Dorsum to plantar surface of the foot with approximately 1 inch (2.5 cm) of the distal tibia-fibula demonstrated; heads of metatarsals superimposed

Exposure
- Optimal image receptor exposure and contrast; no motion.
- Soft tissue, cortical margins, and sharp bony trabeculation clearly demonstrated

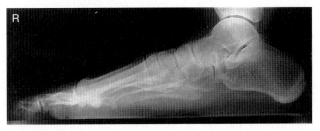

Fig. 4.22 Lateral weight-bearing foot.

Plantodorsal (Axial): Calcaneus

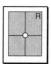

- 8 × 10 inches (18 × 24 cm), portrait
- Nongrid (detail screens)
- Lead masking with multiple exposures on same IR

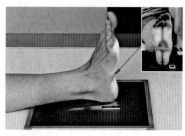

Fig. 4.23 CR 40° to long axis of foot.

Position

- Patient should be supine or seated, with dorsiflex foot so that plantar surface is near perpendicular to IR. If possible, have patient pull on gauze as shown (this may be painful for patient to maintain, so move quickly).
- Center CR to part, with IR centered to projected CR.
- **Dorsoplantar (axial) weight-bearing:** Place patient in the standing upright position with weight placed on affected foot.

Central Ray CR angled 40° to long axis of plantar surface (may require more than 40° from vertical if foot is not dorsiflexed a full 90°):

- CR centered to base of third metatarsal, to emerge just distal and inferior to ankle joint
- **Note 1:** It is important to place the calcaneus on the lower aspect of the IR closest to the x-ray tube due to severe CR angulation.
- **Note 2:** Dorsoplantar (axial) weight-bearing projection, angle the CR 45 degrees anteriorly and directed through the posterior surface of flexed ankle (see fig. 4.26).

SID: 40 inches (100 cm)

Collimation Field Size: Collimate on four sides to area of interest to include soft tissue margins.

kVp Range:					65–75		
	cm	kVp	mA	Time	mAs	SID	Exposure Indicator
S							
M							
L							

Textbook, 11th ed, p. 237

Lower Limb

4

Lateral–Mediolateral: Calcaneus

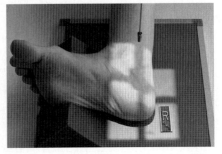
Fig. 4.24 Lateral calcaneus.

- 8 × 10 inches (18 × 24 cm), portrait
- Nongrid
- Lead masking with multiple exposures on same IR

Position
- Patient should be recumbent, on affected side, knee flexed about 45° with unaffected limb behind patient to prevent over-rotation.
- Place support under knee and leg, as needed, for a true lateral.
- Dorsiflex foot so that the plantar surface is near 90° to leg, if possible.

Central Ray: CR ⊥ to midcalcaneus, 1 inch (2.5 cm) inferior to medial malleolus

SID: 40 inches (100 cm)

Collimation Field Size: Collimate on four sides to area of interest; include ankle joint at upper margin and soft tissue margins.

	cm	kVp	mA	Time	mAs	SID	Exposure Indicator
kVp Range:			60–75				
S							
M							
L							

Textbook, 11th ed, p. 238

Plantodorsal and Dorsoplantar (Axial)– Mediolateral: Calcaneus

Evaluation Criteria

Anatomy Demonstrated

- **Plantodorsal and Dorsoplantar-Weight-bearing:** Entire calcaneus from tuberosity to talocalcaneal joint
- **Lateral:** Calcaneus in profile with talus to distal tibia-fibula demonstrated superiorly, navicular and open joint space of the calcaneus and cuboid demonstrated distally

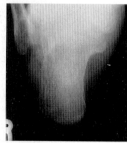

Fig. 4.25 Plantodorsal (axial) calcaneus.

Position

- **Plantodorsal and Dorsoplantar-Weight-bearing:** No rotation with sustentaculum tali in profile medially, open talocalcaneal joint space, no distortion of the calcaneal tuberosity, and adequate elongation of the calcaneus
- **Lateral:** Partial superimposed talus and open talocalcaneal joint. Tarsal sinus and calcaneocuboid joint space should appear open.

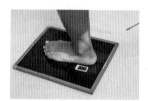

Fig. 4.26 Dorsoplantar (axial) weight-bearing calcaneus.

Exposure

- Optimal image receptor exposure and contrast sufficient to faintly visualize distal fibula through talus; no motion
- Sharp bony margins and trabeculation clearly demonstrated

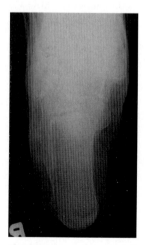

Fig. 4.27 Dorsoplantar (axial) weight-bearing calcaneus.

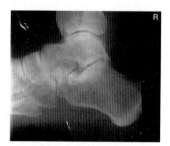

Fig. 4.28 Mediolateral calcaneus.

AP: Ankle

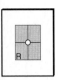

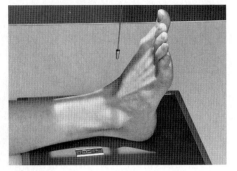

Fig. 4.29 AP ankle.

- 10 × 12 inches (24 × 30 cm), portrait
- Nongrid
- Lead masking with multiple exposures on same IR

Position

- Patient should be supine or seated on table, leg extended, support under knee.
- Center and align leg and ankle joint parallel to edge of IR.
- True AP, ensure no rotation of lower leg, long axis of foot is vertical, parallel to CR.

Central Ray: CR ⊥ to midway between malleoli

SID: 40 inches (100 cm)

Collimation Field Size: Collimate on four sides to area of interest. Include proximal half of metatarsals and distal tibia-fibula and soft tissue margins.

	cm	kVp	mA	Time	mAs	SID	Exposure Indicator
S							
M							
L							

kVp Range: 60–75

Textbook, 11th ed, p. 240

AP Mortise: Ankle

This is a frontal view of the entire ankle mortise joint and should not be a substitute for the routine AP or 45° oblique ankle:

- 10 × 12 inches (24 × 30 cm), portrait
- Nongrid
- Lead masking with multiple exposures on same IR

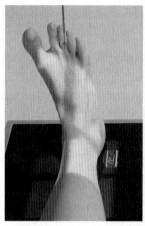

Fig. 4.30 AP, to visualize ankle mortise (15°–20° medial rotation).

Position

- Patient should be supine or seated on table, leg extended, support under knee.
- Center and align ankle joint to CR and to long-axis portion of IR.
- Rotate leg and long axis of foot internally 15°–20° so that **intermalleolar plane is parallel to the IR**.

Central Ray: CR ⊥ to midway between malleoli

SID: 40 inches (100 cm)

Collimation Field Size: Collimate on four sides to area of interest. Include distal tibia-fibula, proximal metatarsals, and soft tissue margins.

Note: The base of the fifth metatarsal is a common fracture site and may be demonstrated in this projection.

	cm	kVp	mA	Time	mAs	SID	Exposure Indicator
S							
M							
L							

kVp Range: 60–75

Textbook, 11th ed, p. 241

AP Oblique—45° Medial Rotation: Ankle

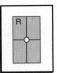

- 10 × 12 inches (24 × 30 cm), portrait
- Nongrid
- Lead masking with multiple exposures on same IR

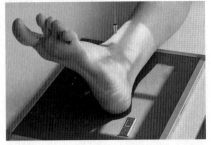

Fig. 4.31 45° AP medial oblique ankle.

Position

- Patient should be supine or seated, leg extended, support under knee.
- Center and align ankle joint to CR and to long axis of IR.
- Rotate leg and foot 45° medially (long axis of foot is 45° to IR).

Central Ray: CR ⊥ to midway between the malleoli

SID: 40 inches (100 cm)

Collimation Field Size: Collimate on four sides to area of interest; include proximal metatarsals, distal tibia-fibula, and soft tissue margins.

Note: The base of the fifth metatarsal is a common fracture site and may be visualized on oblique ankle projections.

	cm	kVp	mA	Time	mAs	SID	Exposure Indicator
S							
M							
L							

kVp Range: 60–75

Textbook, 11th ed, p. 242

AP, AP Mortise, and AP Oblique—45° Medial Rotation: Ankle

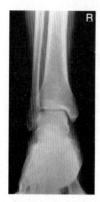

Fig. 4.32 AP ankle. (Courtesy E. Frank, RT[R], FASRT.)

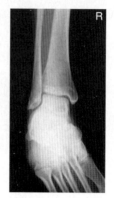

Fig. 4.33 AP mortise ankle.

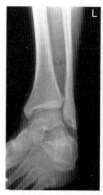

Fig. 4.34 45° AP medial oblique.

Evaluation Criteria

Anatomy Demonstrated

- **AP:** Distal one-third of tibia-fibula, lateral and medial malleoli, talus, and proximal half of metatarsals
- **AP Mortise:** Entire ankle mortise should be open with distal one-third of tibia and fibula, lateral and medial malleoli, talus and proximal half of metatarsals
- **AP 45° Oblique:** Distal one-third of tibia and fibula, malleoli, talus, and proximal half of metatarsals

Position

- **AP:** No rotation with medial mortise joint open and lateral mortise closed
- **AP Mortise:** Open lateral and medial mortise joint surfaces; malleoli in profile
- **AP 45° Oblique:** Distal tibiofibular joint, talus, and medial malleolus open with no or only slight superimposition

Exposure

- Optimal image receptor exposure and contrast sufficient to faintly visualize distal fibula through talus; no motion
- Soft tissue structures, bony margins, and sharp bony trabeculation clearly demonstrated

4

Lower Limb

134

Lateral–Mediolateral or Lateromedial: Ankle

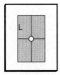

- 10 × 12 inches (24 × 30 cm), portrait
- Nongrid (detail screens)
- Lead masking with multiple exposures on same IR

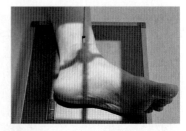

Fig. 4.35 Mediolateral ankle.

Position

- Patient should be recumbent, affected side down, affected knee flexed approximately 45°; place opposite leg behind injured limb to prevent over-rotation.

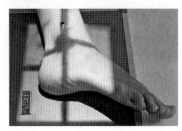

Fig. 4.36 Lateromedial ankle.

- Dorsiflex foot 90° to leg if patient can tolerate it.
- Place support under knee as needed for **true lateral** of foot and ankle.

Central Ray: CR ⊥ to medial malleolus

Note: May also be taken as a lateromedial projection if patient condition allows; may be easier to achieve a **true lateral**

SID: 40 inches (100 cm)

Collimation Field Size: Collimate on four sides to area of interest; include distal tibia and fibula, proximal metatarsals, and soft tissue margins.

	cm	kVp	mA	Time	mAs	SID	Exposure Indicator
kVp Range:				60–75			
S							
M							
L							

Textbook, 11th ed, p. 243

4

Lower Limb

Mediolateral: Ankle

Evaluation Criteria

Anatomy Demonstrated

- Distal one-third of tibia and fibula with lateral view of tarsals, base of fifth metatarsal, navicular and cuboid

Position

- True lateral with no rotation, distal fibula superimposed **over posterior half of tibia**
- Tibiotalar joint open

Exposure

- Optimal image receptor exposure and contrast sufficient to faintly visualize distal fibula through talus; no motion
- Sharp bony margins and trabeculation clearly demonstrated

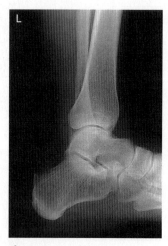

Fig. 4.37 Mediolateral ankle.

AP Stress: Ankle
Inversion and Eversion Positions

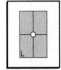

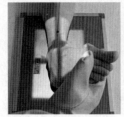

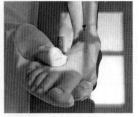

Fig. 4.38 Inversion stress. **Fig. 4.39** Eversion stress.

4

Warning
- Proceed with utmost care with injured patient.
- 10 × 12 inches (24 × 30 cm), portrait or 14 × 17 inches (35 × 43 cm), portrait landscape
- Nongrid
- Lead masking with multiple exposures on same IR

Position
- Patient should be supine or seated on table, leg extended.
- Center and align ankle joint to CR and to long axis of IR.
- Without rotating leg or ankle (true AP), stress is applied to ankle joint by first turning plantar surface of foot inward (inversion stress), then outward (eversion stress).

Central Ray: CR ⊥ to midway between malleoli

SID: 40 inches (100 cm)

Collimation Field Size: Collimate on four sides to area of interest, including proximal metatarsals, distal tibia-fibula, and soft tissue margins.

Lower Limb

	cm	kVp	mA	Time	mAs	SID	Exposure Indicator
kVp Range:					60–75		
S							
M							
L							

Textbook, 11th ed, p. 244

AP: Lower Leg (Tibia-Fibula)

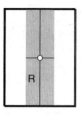

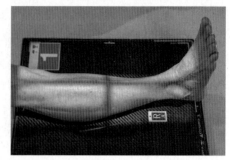

Fig. 4.40 AP lower leg.

- 14 × 17 inches (35 × 43 cm), portrait diagonal IR alignment or two separate IRs to include both joints
- Nongrid
- To make best use of anode heel effect, place knee at cathode end of x-ray beam.

Position

- Patient should be supine, leg extended; ensure no rotation of knee, lower leg, or ankle.
- Include 1 to 2 inches (3 to 5 cm) minimum beyond knee and ankle joints.
- If limb is too long, place the lower leg diagonally (corner to corner) on one 14 × 17-inch (35 × 43 cm) IR to ensure that both joints are included. (Also, if needed, a second, smaller IR may be taken of the joint farthest from the injury site.)

Central Ray: CR ⊥ to midpoint of lower leg (to mid-IR)

SID: Minimum SID of 40 inches (100 cm); may increase to 44–48 inches (110–120 cm)

Collimation Field Size: Collimate on four sides to area of interest; include knee and ankle joints and soft tissue margins.

	cm	kVp	mA	Time	mAs	SID	Exposure Indicator
kVp Range:					70–80		
S							
M							
L							

Textbook, 11th ed, p. 245

Mediolateral: Lower Leg (Tibia-Fibula)

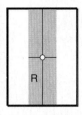

- 14 × 17 inches (35 × 43 cm), portrait; diagonal IR align-

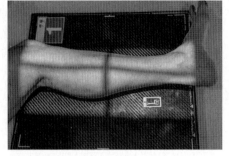

Fig. 4.41 Mediolateral lower leg.

ment or two separate IRs to include both joints
- Nongrid
- To make best use of anode heel effect, place knee at cathode end of x-ray beam.

Position

- Patient should be recumbent, affected side down.
- Place the unaffected limb behind patient to prevent over-rotation.
- Place support under distal portion of the affected foot as needed to ensure a **true lateral** position of foot, ankle, and knee.
- Ensure that both ankle and knee joints are 1–2 inches (3–5 cm) from ends of IR.
- If limb is too long, place the lower leg diagonally (corner to corner) on one 14 × 17-inch (35 × 43 cm) IR to ensure that both joints are included. (Also, if needed, a second, smaller IR may be taken of the joint farthest from the injury site.)

Central Ray: CR ⊥ to midpoint of lower leg (to mid-IR)
SID: Minimum SID of 40 inches (100 cm); may increase to 44–48 inches (110–120 cm)
Collimation Field Size: Collimate on four sides to area of interest; include knee and ankle joints and soft tissue margins.

kVp Range:					65–80	
	cm	kVp	mA	Time	mAs	SID	Exposure Indicator
S							
M							
L							

Textbook, 11th ed, p. 246

AP and Lateral: Lower Leg (Tibia-Fibula)

Evaluation Criteria

Anatomy Demonstrated
- **AP:** Entire tibia-fibula with ankle and knee joints
- **Lateral:** Entire tibia-fibula with ankle and knee joints

Position:
AP
- No rotation, with femoral and tibial condyles in profile
- Knee and ankle joints demonstrated
- Slight overlap at both proximal and distal tibiofibular joints

Lateral
- Ensure that leg is in true lateral position (plane of patella should be perpendicular to IR).
- Knee and ankle joints demonstrated.
- Tibial tuberosity should be in profile.
- Distal fibula overlaps posterior portion of tibia.

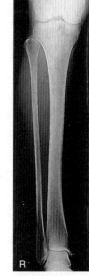

Fig. 4.42 AP lower leg. (Courtesy J. Sanderson, RT.)

Exposure
- Optimal image receptor exposure and contrast; no motion
- Soft tissue and sharp bony trabeculation clearly demonstrated

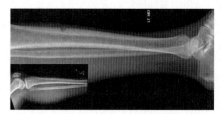

Fig. 4.43 Mediolateral lower leg (proximal and distal).

AP: Knee

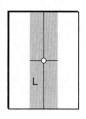

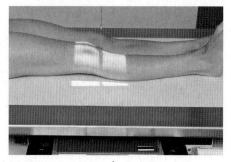

- 10 × 12 inches (24 × 30 cm), portrait
- Grid > 4 inches (10 cm)

Fig. 4.44 AP knee (CR ⊥ to film for average patient).

Position

- Patient should be supine, or seated on table, with leg extended and centered to CR and midline of table or IR.
- Rotate leg slightly internally 3° to 5° for true AP knee (or until **interepicondylar line is parallel** to plane of IR).
- Align and center IR to CR.

Central Ray: CR centered to 1/2 inch (1.25 cm) distal to apex of patella

CR Parallel to Articular Facets (Tibial Plateau). Measure distance from ASIS to tabletop (TT) to determine CR angle:

- <7.5 inches (19 cm) ASIS to TT, 5° caudad
- 7.5 – 9.5 inches (19–24 cm), 0°, ⊥ IR
- >9.5 inches (24 cm), 5° cephalad

SID: 40 inches (100 cm)

Collimation Field Size: Collimate on four sides to area of interest; include soft tissue margins.

	cm	kVp	mA	Time	mAs	SID	Exposure Indicator
kVp Range:					65–80		
S							
M							
L							

Textbook, 11th ed, p. 247

AP Oblique–Medial and Lateral Rotation: Knee

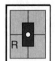
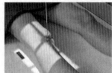
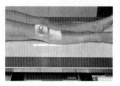

Fig. 4.45 AP 45° medial oblique.

Fig. 4.46 AP 45° lateral oblique.

AP Medial Oblique: Demonstrates fibular head and neck unobscured (Lateral oblique may also be taken.)

AP Lateral Oblique

Demonstrates medial condyles of the femur and tibia in profile:

- 10 × 12 inches (24 × 30 cm), portrait
- Grid > 4 inches (10 cm)

Position

- Patient should be semisupine, leg extended and centered to CR and midline of table.
- Rotate entire leg, including knee, ankle, and foot, internally 45° for medial oblique, and 45° externally for external oblique.
- Center IR to CR.

Central Ray

- CR ⊥ to IR when distance of ASIS to TT is 7.5-9.5 inches (19-24 cm) (see AP Knee)
- CR to midpoint of knee (1/2 inch or 1.25 cm distal to apex of patella)

SID: 40 inches (100 cm)

Collimation Field Size: Collimate on four sides to area of interest; include soft tissue margins.

	cm	kVp	mA	Time	mAs	SID	Exposure Indicator
kVp Range:				65–80			
S							
M							
L							

Textbook, 11th ed, pp. 248 and 249

AP and AP Oblique—Medial and Lateral: Knee

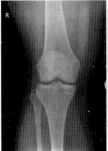 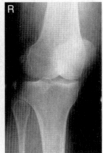 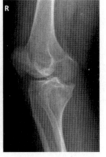

Fig. 4.47 AP knee. (Courtesy Joss Wertz, DO.)

Fig. 4.48 AP medial oblique.

Fig. 4.49 AP lateral oblique. (Courtesy Joss Wertz, DO.)

Evaluation Criteria

Anatomy Demonstrated

- **AP:** Open femorotibial joint space
- **AP Medial Oblique:** Open proximal tibiofibular joint; lateral femoral and tibial condyles in profile
- **AP Lateral Oblique:** Medial femoral and tibial condyles in profile

Position

- **AP:** No rotation is evident by symmetric appearance of femoral and tibial condyles. Medial half of fibular head is superimposed by tibia. Intercondylar eminence is seen.
- **AP Medial Oblique:** Proximal tibiofibular joint is open; tibial lateral condyles are demonstrated. Head and neck of fibula and half of patella are seen without superimposition.
- **AP Lateral Oblique:** Proximal fibula is superimposed by proximal tibia. Medial condyles of femur and tibia are in profile. Approximately half of patella should be seen free of superimposition by the femur.

Exposure

- Optimal image receptor exposure and contrast; outline of patella through distal femur; no motion
- Soft tissue and sharp bony trabeculation clearly demonstrated

Lateral–Mediolateral: Knee

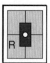

- 8 × 10 inches (18 × 24 cm) or 10 × 12 inches (24 × 30 cm), portrait
- Grid > 4 inches (10 cm)

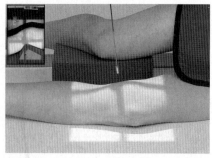

Fig. 4.50 Mediolateral knee, CR 5° cephalad.

Position

- This position may be taken as a horizontal beam lateral or in the lateral recumbent position.
- For patients who are able to flex knee ≈20°–30°, position patient on the affected side, centered to CR and midline of table or IR.
- Unaffected leg and knee are placed behind the patient to prevent over-rotation.
- For patients who are unable to flex the knee because of pain or trauma, use a horizontal beam with IR placed beside knee.
- Place support under affected ankle and foot, if needed, and adjust body rotation as required for a true lateral of knee.
- Align and center IR to CR.

Central Ray

- CR angled 5°–7° cephalad (if lower leg can be elevated to plane of femur, a perpendicular CR can be used)
- CR centered to ≈1 inch (2.5 cm) distal to medial epicondyle

SID: 40 inches (100 cm)

Collimation Field Size: Collimate on four sides to area of interest; include soft tissue margins.

	cm	kVp	mA	Time	mAs	SID	Exposure Indicator
kVp Range:						65–80	
S							
M							
L							

Textbook, 11th ed, p. 250

Lateral–Mediolateral: Knee

Evaluation Criteria

Anatomy Demonstrated

- Distal femur, proximal tibia and fibula, and patella in lateral profile
- Patellofemoral and knee joints open

Position

- True lateral with no rotation; femoral condyles superimposed
- Patella in profile and patellofemoral joint open

Exposure

- Optimal image receptor exposure and contrast; no motion
- Soft tissue (fat pads) and sharp bony trabeculation clearly demonstrated

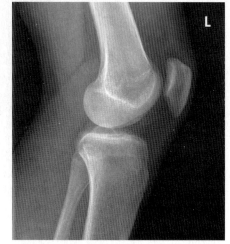

Fig. 4.51 Mediolateral knee.

4

Lower Limb

AP or PA Weight-Bearing Bilateral: Knee

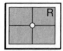

- 14 × 17 inches (35 × 43 cm), landscape
- Grid

Position

AP

- Patient should be erect, standing on step stool or footboard as needed (high enough to lower x-ray tube for horizontal beam).

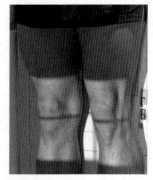

Fig. 4.52 AP weight-bearing—bilateral, CR ⊥ to IR.

- Feet should be straight ahead, knees straight, weight distributed evenly on both feet. Provide support handles for patient stability.

Alternative PA: Patient facing the table or IR holder, with knees against table or vertical IR holder, knees flexed ≈20°

Central Ray: CR ⊥ to midpoint between knee joints, at level of ≈1/2 inch (1.25 cm) distal to apex of patellae

AP: CR horizontal, ⊥ to IR on average patient (see AP Knee)

PA: CR 10° caudad (if knees are flexed ≈20°)

SID: 40 inches (100 cm)

Collimation Field Size: Collimate on four sides to area of interest; include distal femurs, proximal tibia and fibula, and soft tissue margins.

	cm	kVp	mA	Time	mAs	SID	Exposure Indicator
S							
M							
L							

kVp Range: 70–80

Textbook, 11th ed, p. 251

PA Axial Weight-Bearing Bilateral: Knee
Rosenberg Method

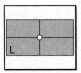

- 14 × 17 inches (35 × 43 cm), landscape
- Grid

Position

- Patient erect PA, standing on attached step of x-ray table or on step stool if the upright bucky is used so that patient is placed high enough for 10° caudad angle
- Weight evenly distributed
- Position feet straight ahead with weight evenly distributed on both feet and knees flexed to 45°; have patient use bucky device for support, with patella touching the upright bucky.
- Align and center bilateral legs and knees to CR and to midline of upright bucky and IR; IR height is adjusted to CR.

Fig. 4.53 PA axial weight-bearing—CR 10° caudad.

Central Ray
- 10° caudad to midpoint between knee joints— 1/2 inch (1.25 cm) below apex of patella

SID: 40 inches (100 cm)

Collimation Field Size: Collimate on four sides to area of interest; include distal femora, proximal tibia, and soft tissue margins.

	cm	kVp	mA	Time	mAs	SID	Exposure Indicator
kVp Range:				70–80			
S							
M							
L							

Textbook, 11th ed, p. 252

4

Lower Limb

AP or PA Weight-Bearing Bilateral: Knee
Rosenberg Method

Evaluation Criteria

Anatomy Demonstrated

- Distal femur, proximal tibia and fibula, and femorotibial joint spaces

Position

- No rotation of both knees evident by symmetric appearance of joint spaces

Exposure

- Optimal image receptor exposure and contrast; no motion

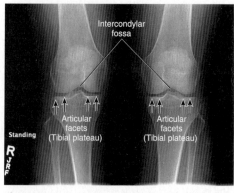

Fig. 4.54 AP Weight-bearing knee—bilateral.

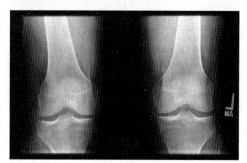

Fig. 4.55 PA axial weight-bearing knees—Rosenberg method.

- Sharp bony trabeculation clearly demonstrated

PA and AP Axial ("Tunnel Views"): Intercondylar Fossa
Camp Coventry and Holmblad Methods

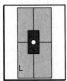

- 8 × 10 inches (18 × 24 cm), portrait, or 14 × 17 inches (35 × 43 cm) for bilateral studies, portrait
- Grid

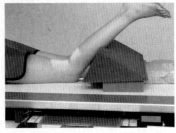

Fig. 4.56 PA axial projection (Camp Coventry).

Position

- Camp Coventry method: Patient prone, knee flexed 40°–50°, large support under ankle
- Holmblad method: Patient kneeling on x-ray table or partially standing (requires elevation of examination table)
- Knee centered to CR
- IR centered to projected CR

Fig. 4.57 Alternative Holmblad method—patient kneeling, leans forward 20°–30° – CR ⊥ to IR.

Central Ray

- **Camp Coventry method:** CR 40°–50° caudad (⊥ to lower leg), centered to knee joint, to emerge at distal margin of patella
- **Holmblad method:** CR ⊥ to lower leg to midpopliteal crease

SID: 40 inches (100 cm)

Collimation Field Size: Collimate on four sides to area of interest; include soft tissue margins.

	cm	kVp	mA	Time	mAs	SID	Exposure Indicator
kVp Range:					70–80		
S							
M							
L							

PA: Patella

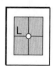

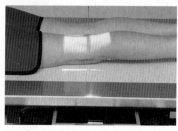

- 8 × 10 inches (18 × 24 cm), portrait
- Grid

Fig. 4.58 PA patella.

Position

- Patient should be prone, knee centered to CR and midline of table or IR.
- If patella area is painful, place pad under thigh and leg to prevent direct pressure on patella.
- Rotate anterior knee approximately 5° internally, or as needed, to place an imaginary line between the epicondyles parallel to the plane of the IR for true PA.
- Align and center IR to CR.

Central Ray: CR ⊥, centered to midpatella area (at midpopliteal crease)

SID: 40 inches (100 cm)

Collimation Field Size: Collimate on four sides to area of interest; include soft tissue margins.

	cm	kVp	mA	Time	mAs	SID	Exposure Indicator
S							
M							
L							

kVp Range: 70–80

Textbook, 11th ed, p. 257

Lateral–Mediolateral: Patella

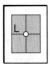

- 8 × 10 inches (18 × 24 cm), portrait
- Grid > 4 inches (10 cm)

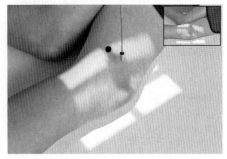

Fig. 4.59 Mediolateral patella.

Position

- Patient recumbent on affected side, opposite knee, and leg behind patient to prevent over-rotation
- Knee flexed only 5°–10° to prevent separation of fractured fragments, if present
- Patellofemoral joint area centered to CR and midline of IR

Central Ray: CR ⊥, centered to midpatellofemoral joint

SID: 40 inches (100 cm)

Collimation Field Size: Collimate on four sides to area of interest; include soft tissue margins.

	cm	kVp	mA	Time	mAs	SID	Exposure Indicator
S							
M							
L							

kVp Range: 70–80

Textbook, 11th ed, p. 258

PA Axial: Intercondylar Fossa and Patella

Evaluation Criteria

Anatomy Demonstrated
- **PA Axial:** Intercondylar fossa, femoral condyles, tibial plateaus, and intercondylar eminence
- **PA:** Knee joint and patella outline through distal femur
- **Lateral:** Patella, patellofemoral joint, and femorotibial joint demonstrated in profile

Position
- **PA Axial:** No rotation evidenced by symmetric distal femoral condyles and intercondylar eminence centered
- **PA:** No rotation, femoral condyles appear symmetric; patella appears centered to femur
- **Lateral:** Patella in profile and patellofemoral joint open

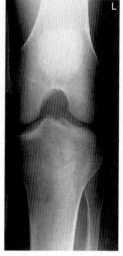

Fig. 4.60 PA axial—intercondylar fossa projection.

Exposure
- Optimal image receptor exposure and contrast; no motion
- Soft tissue and sharp bony trabeculation clearly demonstrated

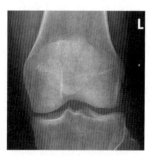

Fig. 4.61 PA patella. (Courtesy Joss Wertz, DO.)

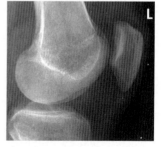

Fig. 4.62 Lateral patella.

Tangential–Axial: Patella

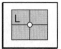

Merchant Bilateral Method

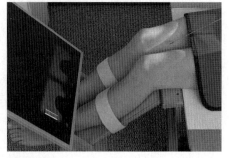

Fig. 4.63 Bilateral tangential (Merchant method).

- 8 × 10 inches (18 × 24 cm), landscape or 14 × 17 inches (35 × 43 cm) for bilateral studies; landscape
- Nongrid
- Adjustable leg and IR-holding device required

Position

- Patient should be supine with knees flexed 40° on leg supports (important for patient to be comfortable with legs completely relaxed to prevent patellae from being drawn into intercondylar sulcus).
- Place IR on supports against legs about 12 inches (30 cm) distal to patellae, perpendicular to CR.

Central Ray
- CR 30° caudad from horizontal (30° from long axis of femora)
- CR to midway between patellae

SID: 48–72 inches (120–180 cm) (increased SID reduces magnification)

Collimation Field Size: Collimate on four sides to area of interest; include soft tissue margins.

	cm	kVp	mA	Time	mAs	SID	Exposure Indicator
kVp Range:				70–80			
S							
M							
L							

Textbook, 11th ed, p. 259

Tangential–Axial (Prone): Patella
Hughston and Settegast Methods

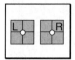

Generally performed bilaterally for comparison purposes:

- 14 × 17 inches (35 × 43 cm), landscape for bilateral study; 10 × 12 inches (24 × 30 cm), landscape for unilateral
- Nongrid
- Lead masking with multiple exposures on same IR

Position

- **Hughston:** Patient prone, knee flexed between 50° and 60° from full extension
- Patient may use gauze or tape to hold leg in position; may support foot on supporting device (not collimator).
- **Settegast:** Patient prone, knee flexed 90°

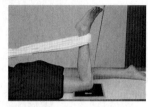

Fig. 4.64 Settegast—knee flexed 90° – CR 15°–20° to lower leg.

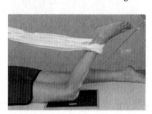

Fig. 4.65 Hughston—knee flexed 50°–60° – CR 45° cephalad. Warning: Possible hot collimator, use pad.

Central Ray: CR centered to midpatellofemoral joint

Hughston: CR 45° cephalad (CR tangential to patellofemoral joint space) (knee flexed 50°–60°)

Settegast:

Warning: This acute flexion of the knee should not be attempted until fracture of the patella has been ruled out by other projections.

CR 15°–20° cephalad (CR tangential to patellofemoral joint space) (knee flexed 90°)

SID: 40–48 inches (100–120 cm)

Collimate: Collimate on four sides to area of interest; include soft tissue margins.

	cm	kVp	mA	Time	mAs	SID	Exposure Indicator
kVp Range:					70–80		
S							
M							
L							

Textbook, 11th ed, pp. 260 and 261

Superoinferior Sitting Tangential: Patella
Hobbs Modification

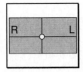

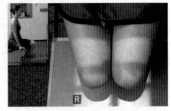

Fig. 4.66 Tangential superoinferior (Hobbs modification).

Warning: This acute flexion of the knee should not be attempted until fracture of the patella has been ruled out by other projections.

Generally performed bilaterally on one IR for comparison purposes
- 14 × 17 inches (35 × 43 cm), landscape or 8 × 10 inches (18 × 24 cm), landscape (unilateral)
- Nongrid

Position
- Patient seated in chair, IR placed under knees resting on a step stool or support to help reduce OID
- Knees flexed with feet placed slightly underneath chair

Central Ray: Perpendicular to IR (tangential to patellofemoral joint) centered to midpatellofemoral joints

SID: 48–50 inches (120–125 cm)

Collimation Field Size: Collimate on four sides to area of interest; include distal femora, patella and soft tissue margins.

	cm	kVp	mA	Time	mAs	SID	Exposure Indicator
kVp Range:					70–80		
S							
M							
L							

Textbook, 11th ed, p. 262

4

Lower Limb

Superoinferior Sitting Tangential (Bilateral): Patella
Hobbs Modification

Evaluation Criteria

Anatomy Demonstrated

- Tangential view of patella
- Patellofemoral joint space open

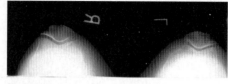

Fig. 4.67 Superoinferior tangential sitting method.

Position

- Separation of patella and intercondylar sulcus
- Patellofemoral joint open

Exposure

- Optimal image receptor exposure and contrast; no motion
- Soft tissue and sharp bony trabeculation clearly demonstrated

AP: Lower Limb (Pediatric)

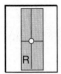

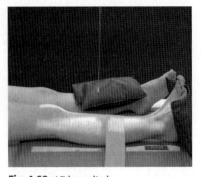

Fig. 4.68 AP lower limb.

- IR size and placement—determined by size of body part, portrait frequently
- Nongrid
- Shield radiosensitive tissues outside region of interest. Follow local regulations, department policy, and protocol in the use of shielding.

Note: If the foot is the specific area of interest, AP and lateral projections of the foot only may be required.

Position: Patient Supine, Include Entire Limb

- A second IR of pelvis or proximal femur may be required (see Chapter 16 of the textbook).
- Immobilization techniques should be used when necessary.
- Use parental assistance only if necessary; provide lead gloves and apron.

Central Ray: CR ⊥, centered to midlimb (mid-IR)

Minimum SID: 40 inches (100 cm)

Collimation Field Size: Collimate on four sides to area of interest; include soft tissue margins.

	cm	kVp	mA	Time	mAs	SID	Exposure Indicator
kVp Range:					50–60		
S							
M							
L							

Textbook, 11th ed, p. 646

4

Lower Limb

Lateral: Lower Limb (Pediatric)

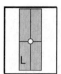

- IR size and placement determined by size of body part, portrait frequently
- Nongrid
- Shield radiosensitive tissues outside region of interest.
Follow local regulations, department policy, and protocol in the use of shielding.

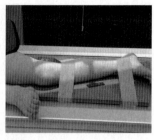

Fig. 4.69 Lateral lower limb (see *Note*).

Note: If the foot is the specific area of interest, AP and lateral projections of the foot only may a be required.

Position
- Patient should be semisupine, include entire limb.
- Immobilization techniques should be used when necessary. Abduct (frog leg) affected limb into lateral position, and immobilize with tape or compression band (do not attempt in patients with hip trauma or hip disease).
- Bilateral examinations may be requested on one IR for a bone survey or for comparison purposes.
- If parental assistance is necessary, provide lead gloves and apron.

Central Ray: CR ⊥, centered to midlimb (mid-IR)
Minimum SID: 40 inches (100 cm)
Collimation Field Size: Collimate on four sides to area of interest; include soft tissue margins.

kVp Range:					50–60	
	cm	kVp	mA	Time	mAs	SID	Exposure Indicator
S							
M							
L							

Textbook, 11th ed, p. 646

AP and Mediolateral: Foot (Pediatric)

Congenital Clubfoot—Kite Method

- 8 × 10 inches (18 × 24 cm), portrait
- Nongrid

Fig. 4.70
AP foot (Kite method).

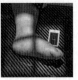

Fig. 4.71
Mediolateral foot (Kite method).

Note: With the **Kite method**, no attempt is made to straighten the foot when placing it on IR. The foot is held or immobilized for AP and lateral projections 90° from each other. Both feet are generally imaged for comparison.

Position

- **AP:** Elevate patient on support, flex knee, foot on IR.
- **Lateral:** Patient or leg on side, affected side down; use tape or compression band.

Central Ray

- **AP:** CR ⊥ to IR, directed to midtarsals (Kite recommends no angle)
- **Lateral:** CR ⊥, centered to proximal metatarsal area

Minimum SID: 40 inches (100 cm)

Collimation Field Size: Collimate on four sides to area of interest; include soft tissue margins.

kVp Range:				50–60			
	cm	kVp	mA	Time	mAs	SID	Exposure Indicator
S							
M							
L							

Textbook, 11th ed, p. 646

4

Lower Limb

Femur and Pelvis

(R) Routine, (S) Special

Radiation Protection

- Exposure factor selection should be optimized in accordance with ALARA.
- Collimate on four sides to anatomy of interest when feasible.

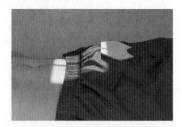

Fig. 5.1 Male gonadal shielding.

Accurate gonadal shielding for pelvis and hip examinations is especially critical due to the proximity of radiation-sensitive tissues (proximal femurs, gonads, noninvolved portions of the pelvis) to the primary x-ray beam. However, shielding must not interfere with the clinical intent of radiographic study. Radiologic technologists should follow local regulations, department policy and protocol in the use of shielding.

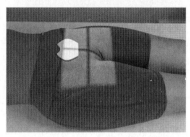

Fig. 5.2 Female ovarian shielding (superior borders at or slightly above level of ASISs and lower border just above pubis).

Digital Imaging Considerations

- A higher kVp range (80 to 90) with lower mAs may be used for examinations of the hips and pelvis of adults to reduce the total radiation dose to the patient.
- Close collimation to the area of interest is important for all procedures, including the hips and pelvis.
- **Accurate centering:** The body part and the central ray (CR) should be centered to the IR.
- Anatomy thickness and kVp range are deciding factors for whether a grid is to be used. Virtual grid technology may eliminate the need for a physical grid
- See Appendix A for reducing patient dose.

Localization Methods for Femoral Head and Neck

First Method: Location of the femoral head and neck regions can be accurately determined by first drawing an imaginary line between two landmarks, the **ASIS** and the **symphysis pubis**. The midpoint of this line is determined, from which a perpendicular imaginary line is drawn to locate the head or neck. The femoral head (A) is approximately 1.5 inches (4 cm) down on this line. The midfemoral neck (B) is approximately 2.5 inches (6–7 cm) down, as shown in Fig. 5.3.

Second Method: A second method for locating the femoral neck (B) is ≈1–2 inches (2.5–5 cm) medial to the ASIS at the level of the proximal or upper margin of the symphysis pubis, which is 3–4 inches (8–10 cm) distal to the ASIS.

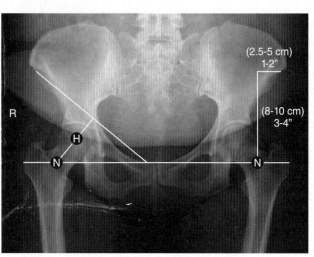

Fig. 5.3 H, Femoral head. N, Femoral neck.

AP: Femur

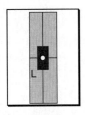

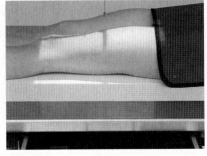

Fig. 5.4 AP mid- and distal femur.

- 14 × 17 inches (35 × 43 cm), portrait
- Grid
- Due to the anode heel effect, place hip at cathode end of x-ray tube. If available, use compensating filter.

Note: For adults, a second, smaller IR of either the hip or the knee should be performed on trauma patients to demonstrate both knee and hip joints to rule out possible fractures.

Position
- Patient should be supine, femur centered to midline of table or grid IR.
- Rotate entire lower limb internally ≈5° for true AP of midfemur and distal femur. Rotate limb internally 15° for true AP of proximal femur, to include hip.
- Lower border of IR ≈2 inches (5 cm) below knee to include knee joint adequately (see AP Unilateral Hip for proximal femur, p. 291 in the textbook).

Central Ray: CR ⊥ to femur, to mid-IR
SID: 40 inches (100 cm)
Collimation Field Size: Collimate on four sides to area of interest to include soft tissue margins.

kVp Range:					75–85	
	cm	kVp	mA	Time	mAs	SID	Exposure Indicator
S							
M							
L							

Textbook, 11th ed, p. 280

Lateral: Femur

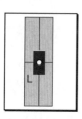

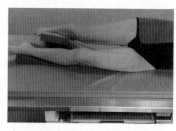

Fig. 5.5 Mediolateral mid- and distal femur.

Warning: Perform with horizontal beam if fracture is suspected.

- 14 × 17 inches (35 × 43 cm), portrait
- Grid
- Due to the anode heel effect, place hip at cathode end of x-ray tube. If available, use compensating filter.

Note: For adults, take a second, smaller IR of lateral hip or lateral knee if both joints are areas of interest.

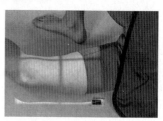

Fig. 5.6 Mediolateral mid- and proximal femur.

Position

- Patient should be lateral recumbent, with unaffected leg placed behind patient to prevent over-rotation.
- Include sufficient amount of either knee or hip at one end of IR.
- Flex affected knee ≈45°, and align femur to midline of table.
- Shield radiosensitive tissues when possible.

Central Ray: CR ⊥ femur, to mid-IR

SID: 40 inches (100 cm)

Collimation Field Size: Long, narrow collimation on four sides to area of interest should include soft tissue margins.

kVp Range:					75–85	
	cm	kVp	mA	Time	mAs	SID	Exposure Indicator
S							
M							
L							

Textbook, 11th ed, p. 281

AP and Lateral: Mid- and Distal Femur

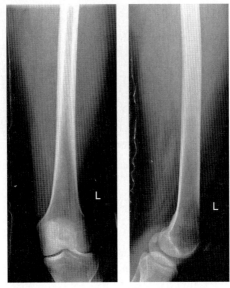

Fig. 5.7 AP.   **Fig. 5.8** Lateral.

Evaluation Criteria

Anatomy Demonstrated

- **AP and Lateral:** Distal two-thirds of femur, including knee joint

Position

- **AP:** No rotation, femoral and tibial condyles appear symmetric in size and shape
- **Lateral:** True lateral, femoral condyles appear superimposed

Exposure:

AP and Lateral

- Optimal image receptor exposure and contrast; no motion
- Fine trabecular markings

Horizontal Beam Lateral: Mid- and Distal Femur (Trauma)

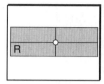

- 14 × 17 inches (35 × 43 cm), portrait (to long axis of femur)
- Portable grid

Note: For proximal femur injuries, perform axiolateral (Danelius-Miller method) hip.

Fig. 5.9 Horizontal beam trauma projection (mid- and distal femur).

Position

- Without moving trauma patient from the supine position, gently lift injured leg, and place support under knee and leg.
- Place vertical IR between legs, as far superiorly as possible, and include knee distally. Use tape to hold grid IR in position.

Central Ray: CR horizontal beam, ⊥ to femur to midpoint of IR
SID: 40 inches (100 cm)
Collimation Field Size: Collimate on four sides to area of interest to include soft tissue margins.

	cm	kVp	mA	Time	mAs	SID	Exposure Indicator
kVp Range:					75–85		
S							
M							
L							

Textbook, 11th ed, p. 281

AP Bilateral: Proximal Femora (Bilateral Hips)

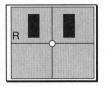

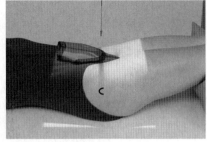

Warning: Do not attempt to rotate legs internally if a hip fracture or dislocation is suspected. Perform position with minimal movement of affected leg.

Fig. 5.10 AP bilateral hips.

Note: For AP pelvis centering, see p. 283 in textbook.

- 14 × 17 inches (35 × 43 cm), landscape
- Grid

Position

- Patient should be erect or supine, aligned and centered to CR and IR, both legs extended and equally rotated internally 15°–20°.
- Ensure no rotation of pelvis (bilateral ASISs the same distances from tabletop). Support under knees for patient comfort.
- Separate legs and feet, then **internally rotate** long axes of feet and entire lower limb **15°–20°**.
- Center IR to CR.

Central Ray: CR ⊥ to midpoint between femoral heads (about 1 inch [2 cm] superior to symphysis pubis and approximately 2 inches [5 cm] inferior to level of ASIS).

SID: 40 inches (100 cm)

Collimation Field Size: Collimate on four sides to area of interest to include soft tissue margins.

Respiration: Suspend during exposure.

	cm	kVp	mA	Time	mAs	SID	Exposure Indicator
kVp Range:					80–90		
S							
M							
L							

Textbook, 11th ed, p. 283

AP Unilateral: Proximal Femur (Hip)

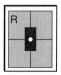

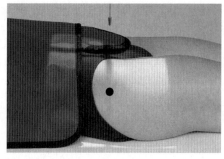

Fig. 5.11 AP hip—CR to femoral neck.

Warning: Do not attempt to rotate legs if fracture is suspected. An AP pelvis projection to include both hips for comparison should be completed before an AP unilateral hip is performed for possible hip or pelvis trauma.

- 10 × 12 inches (24 × 30 cm), portrait
- Grid

Position

- Patient should be erect or supine, leg extended and rotated internally 15°–20° (nontrauma).
- Locate and center femoral neck to CR; support may be placed under knees for patient comfort.
- Ensure **no rotation** of pelvis (equal distance from ASISs to table).
- Rotate affected leg **internally 15°–20°**.
- Center IR to CR

Central Ray: CR ⊥ IR, directed to 1–2 inches (2.5–5 cm) distal to midfemoral neck (to include entire orthopedic appliance of hip, if present)

SID: 40 inches (100 cm)

Collimation Field Size: Collimate on four sides to area of interest to include soft tissue margins.

Respiration: Suspend during exposure.

kVp Range:					80–85		
	cm	kVp	mA	Time	mAs	SID	Exposure Indicator
S							
M							
L							

Textbook, 11th ed, p. 291

5

Femur and Pelvis

AP Unilateral: Proximal Femur (Hip)

Evaluation Criteria

Anatomy Demonstrated
- Proximal one-third of femur and adjacent parts of pelvic girdle
- Any existing orthopedic appliance must be demonstrated in its entirety.

Position
- Greater trochanter, femoral head and neck in profile
- Lesser trochanter not visible or minimally only

Exposure
- Optimal image receptor exposure and contrast; no motion
- Sharp trabecular markings clearly demonstrated

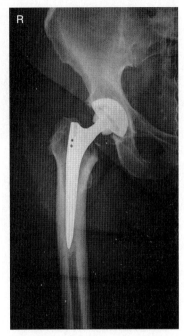

Fig. 5.12 AP hip. (Copyright Getty Images/DieterMeyrl.)

Femur and Pelvis

Unilateral Modified Cleaves Method: Lateral Hip (Nontrauma)

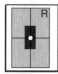

Warning: Do not attempt on patient with destructive hip disease or potential hip fracture or dislocation. This could result in significant displacement of fracture fragments (see lateral trauma projections).

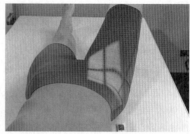

Fig. 5.13 Right hip modified Cleaves lateral (for femoral neck).

- 10 × 12 inches (24 × 30 cm), landscape
- Grid

Position

- Patient should be supine or erect.
- For femoral neck, flex affected knee and hip, and abduct femur 45° from vertical.*

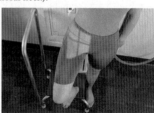

Fig. 5.14 Erect version of modified Cleaves method.

- For femoral head, acetabulum, and proximal femoral shaft, oblique patient 35°–45° toward affected side and abduct leg to tabletop or wall bucky, if possible. Center hip and neck area to CR.
- Center IR to CR.

Central Ray: CR ⊥ to midfemoral neck (see localization methods on p. 275 in the textbook.)

SID: 40 inches (100 cm)

Collimation Field Size: Collimate on four sides to area of interest to include soft tissue margins.

Respiration: Suspend during exposure.

*Less abduction of femora of only 20°–30° from vertical provides for the least foreshortening of femoral neck.

	cm	kVp	mA	Time	mAs	SID	Exposure Indicator
S							
M							
L							

kVp Range: 80–85

Textbook, 11th ed, p. 294

Bilateral Modified Cleaves Method: Hips (Nontrauma)

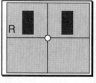

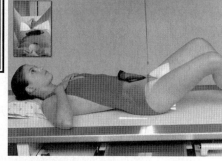

Warning: Do not attempt on patient with destructive hip disease or potential hip fracture or dislocation. This could result in significant

Fig. 5.15 Bilateral modified Cleaves method.

displacement of fracture fragments (see lateral trauma projections).

- 14 × 17 inches (35 × 43 cm), landscape
- Grid

Position

- Patient should be supine, centered to CR and IR; flex hips and knees and **abduct both femora equally** 40°–45° from vertical,* if possible, with plantar surfaces of feet together.
- Ensure **no rotation** of pelvis (ASISs equal distance from table).
- Center IR to CR, **shield radiosensitive tissues** (per department protocol).

Central Ray: CR ⊥ to IR, to level of femoral heads (≈3 inches or 7–8 cm inferior to level of ASIS)

SID: 40 inches (100 cm)

Collimation Field Size: Collimate on four sides to area of interest to include soft tissue margins.

Respiration: Suspend during exposure.

*Less abduction of femora of only 20°–30° from vertical provides for the least foreshortening of femoral neck.

	cm	kVp	mA	Time	mAs	SID	Exposure Indicator
S							
M							
L							

kVp Range: 80–90

Textbook, 11th ed, p. 293

Femur and Pelvis

5

Bilateral Modified Cleaves Method: Hips (Nontrauma)

Evaluation Criteria

Anatomy Demonstrated

- Femoral heads and necks, acetabulum, and trochanteric anatomy

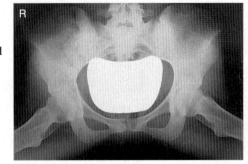

Fig. 5.16 AP bilateral modified Cleaves method.

Position

- No rotation evident by symmetry of pelvic bones
- Lesser trochanters equal in size
- Minimal distortion of femoral neck
- Greater trochanters superimposed over femoral necks

Exposure

- Optimal image receptor exposure and contrast; no motion
- Sharp trabecular markings clearly demonstrated

Axiolateral Inferosuperior: Lateral Hip (Trauma)
Danelius-Miller Method

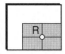

Warning: Do not attempt to rotate leg internally on initial trauma examination.

- 10 × 12 inches (24 × 30 cm), landscape (lengthwise to long axis of femur)
- Portable grid
- If available, use compensating filter.

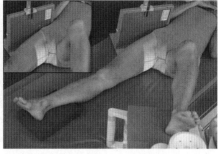

Fig. 5.17 Axiolateral trauma hip (pad under foot).

Position
- Patient should be supine, no rotation of pelvis.
- Flex and elevate unaffected knee and hip, and provide support.
- Rotate affected leg internally 15° **unless contraindicated by possible hip fracture**.
- Place IR in the crease above iliac crest, and adjust so that it is **parallel to femoral neck** and **perpendicular to CR**. Use IR holder if available, or use sandbags to hold IR/grid in place.

Central Ray: CR horizontal, perpendicular to femoral neck area and IR (see "hip localization methods" in chapter introduction)

SID: 40 inches (100 cm)

Collimation Field Size: Collimate on four sides to area of interest to include soft tissue margins.

Respiration: Suspend during exposure.

	cm	kVp	mA	Time	mAs	SID	Exposure Indicator
S							
M							
L							

kVp Range: 80–95

Textbook, 11th ed, p. 292

Axiolateral Inferosuperior: Lateral Hip (Trauma)
Danelius-Miller Method

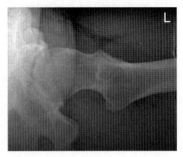

Fig. 5.18 Axiolateral hip.

Evaluation Criteria

Anatomy Demonstrated
- Entire femoral head and neck, trochanters, and acetabulum
- Orthopedic appliance demonstrated in its entirety

Position
- Femoral head, neck, and acetabulum demonstrated with little superimposition of opposite hip
- No grid lines visible on image
- Minimal distortion of femoral neck

Exposure
- Optimal density (brightness) and contrast; no motion
- Sharp trabecular markings clearly seen

AP: Pelvis

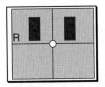

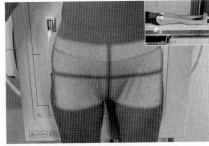

To include proximal femora, pelvic girdle, sacrum, and coccyx

Fig. 5.19 AP pelvis (entire pelvis centered to IR).

Warning: Do not attempt to rotate legs internally if a hip fracture or dislocation is suspected. Perform position with minimal movement of affected leg.
Note: For bilateral hips centering, see p. 283 in the textbook.
- 14 × 17 inches (35 × 43 cm), landscape
- Grid

Position
- Position performed erect or supine; pelvis centered to imaging device, legs extended.
- Both feet, knees, and legs should be equally rotated internally 15°–20° (secure with tape, if necessary). Support under knees for comfort.
- Ensure no rotation of pelvis (ASIS equal distance from TT).
- Center IR to CR (include entire pelvis).

Central Ray: CR ⊥, midway between ASIS and symphysis pubis (approximately 2 inches [5 cm] distal to level of ASIS)
SID: 40 inches (100 cm)
Collimation Field Size: Collimate on four sides to area of interest to include soft tissue margins.
Respiration: Suspend during exposure.

kVp Range:						80–90	
	cm	kVp	mA	Time	mAs	SID	Exposure Indicator
S							
M							
L							

Textbook, 11th ed, p. 283

AP: Pelvis

Evaluation Criteria
Anatomy Demonstrated
- Pelvic girdle, L5, sacrum, coccyx, and proximal femora
- Orthopedic appliance demonstrated in its entirety (if present)

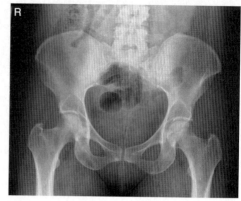

Fig. 5.20 AP pelvis.

Position
- Lesser trochanters generally not visible (nontrauma)
- **No rotation** evident by symmetry of ilia and obturator foramina

Exposure
- Optimal image receptor exposure and contrast visualizing L5 and sacrum and margins of femoral heads and acetabula; no motion
- Soft tissue and sharp trabecular markings clearly demonstrated

AP Axial (Inlet and Outlet): Pelvis

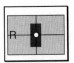

- 14 × 17 inches (35 × 43 cm), landscape
- Grid

Position

- Patient should be supine, align midsagittal plane to CR and to midline of table or IR.
- No rotation of pelvis is necessary (ASISs the same distance from tabletop).
- Center IR to projected CR.
- Gonadal shielding may not be possible without obscuring essential anatomy (per department protocol).

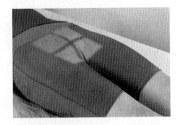

Fig. 5.21 AP axial pelvis.

Fig. 5.22 CR 40° caudal for inlet.

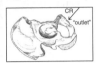

Fig. 5.23 CR cephalad 20°–35° for males and 30°–45° for females—outlet.

Central Ray

- **Inlet:** CR 40° caudal to level of ASISs, male and female
- **Outlet** (Taylor method): CR: male, 20°–35° cephalad; female, 30°–45° cephalad centered 1–2 inches (2.5–5 cm) inferior to symphysis pubis or greater trochanters

SID: 40 inches (100 cm)

Collimation Field Size: Collimate on four sides to area of interest to include soft tissue margins.

Respiration: Suspend during exposure.

	cm	kVp	mA	Time	mAs	SID	Exposure Indicator
kVp Range:					80–90		
S							
M							
L							

Textbook, 11th ed, pp. 284 and 285

AP Axial (Inlet and Outlet): Pelvis

Evaluation Criteria

Anatomy Demonstrated

- **Inlet:** Pelvic ring or inlet in its entirety
- **Outlet:** Superior/inferior rami of pubis and ramus of ischium

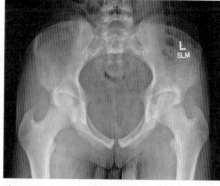

Fig. 5.24 AP axial inlet projection.

Position

- **Inlet:** Ischial spines are demonstrated and equal in size; pelvic ring; no rotation.
- **Outlet:** Obturator foramina are equal in size; anterior/inferior pelvic bones; no rotation

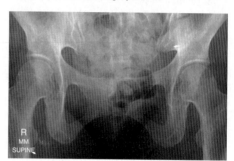

Fig. 5.25 AP axial outlet projection. (Image courtesy Joss Wertz, DO.)

Exposure

- Optimal image receptor exposure and contrast; no motion
- Body and superior rami of pubis demonstrated
- Superimposed anterior and posterior portions of pelvic ring
- Bony margins and trabecular markings appear sharp.

Posterior Oblique: Acetabulum and Pelvic Ring
Judet Method

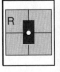

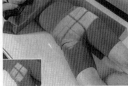

Fig. 5.26 Downside acetabulum.

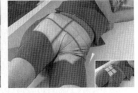

Fig. 5.27 Upside acetabulum.

Note: Both sides are generally imaged for comparison, either both for upside or both for downside.

Pelvic Ring: Possible pelvic ring fractures due to a contrecoup injury, the entire pelvis must be included. In this case, centering should be adjusted to include both hips.

- 10 × 12 inches (24 × 30 cm), portrait, or 14 × 17 inches (35 × 43 cm), landscape (if both hips must be seen on each projection)
- Grid

Position

- Patient should be semisupine or erect in 45° posterior oblique position, centered for either upside or downside hip joint (dependent on anatomy of interest).
- Place 45° support under elevated side, position arms and legs as shown to maintain this position.

Central Ray

- **Downside:** CR ⊥ to 2 inches (5 cm) distal and 2 inches (5 cm) medial to downside ASIS
- **Upside:** CR ⊥ to 2 inches (5 cm) distal to upside ASIS

SID: 40 inches (100 cm)

Collimation Field Size: Collimate on four sides to area of interest to include soft tissue margins.

Respiration: Suspend during exposure.

	cm	kVp	mA	Time	mAs	SID	Exposure Indicator
kVp Range:				80–90			
S							
M							
L							

Femur and Pelvis

Posterior Oblique: Acetabulum
Judet Method

Evaluation Criteria
Anatomy Demonstrated

- **Downside:** Anterior rim of acetabulum, posterior ilioischial column, and iliac wing demonstrated
- **Upside:** Posterior rim of acetabulum, anterior ilioischial column, and obturator foramen demonstrated
- For pelvic ring studies, the entire pelvis must be demonstrated for both oblique positions.

Position

- **Downside:** Iliac wing elongated and obturator foramen closed
- **Upside:** Iliac wing foreshortened and obturator foramen open

Exposure

- Optimal image receptor exposure and contrast; no motion
- Bony margins and trabecular markings are sharp.

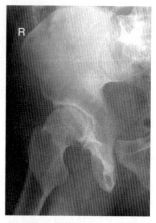
Fig. 5.28 RPO—downside visualized.

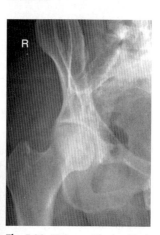
Fig. 5.29 LPO—upside visualized.

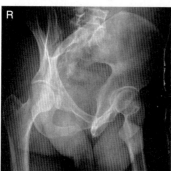
Fig. 5.30 LPO-pelvic ring. (Case courtesy of Dr Luke Danaher, Radiopaedia.org, rID: 39777.)

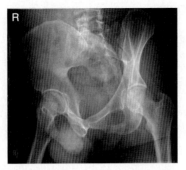

Fig. 5.31 RPO-pelvic ring. (Case courtesy of Dr Luke Danaher, Radiopaedia.org, rID: 39777.)

PA Axial Oblique: Acetabulum
Teufel Method

Both sides are generally imaged for comparison.
- 10 × 12 inches (24 × 30 cm), portrait
- Grid

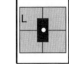

Position
- Patient should be semiprone; affected side down.
- Rotate patient's body 35°–40° anterior oblique.

Central Ray
- CR 12° cephalad
- When anatomy of interest is downside, direct CR ⊥ at 1 inch (2.5 cm) superior to level of greater trochanter; ≈2 inches (5 cm) lateral to the midsagittal plane

SID: 40 inches (100 cm)

Collimation Field Size: Collimate on four sides to area of interest to include soft tissue margins.

	cm	kVp	mA	Time	mAs	SID	Exposure Indicator
kVp Range:					75–85		
S							
M							
L							

Textbook, 11th ed, p. 288

PA Axial Oblique: Acetabulum
Teufel Method

Evaluation Criteria

Anatomy Demonstrated

- Centered to the **downside** acetabulum, superoposterior wall of the acetabulum is demonstrated.

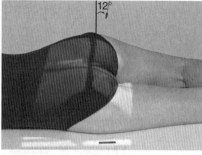

Fig. 5.32 PA axial oblique (Teufel method)

Position

- Fovea capitis with the femoral head in profile
- Obturator foramen open

Exposure

- Optimal image receptor exposure and contrast; no motion
- Bony margins and sharp trabecular markings clearly seen

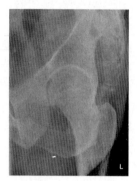

Fig. 5.33 PA axial oblique.

AP Oblique: Acetabulum
False Profile and Modified False Profile Method

- 10 × 12 inches (24 × 30 cm), portrait
- Grid

Position

- Place patient in **posterior oblique**, with both pelvis and thorax rotated **65°** to to the imaging device.
- Rotate dependent lower limb until foot is parallel to IR (see **NOTE**)
- Center IR longitudinally to CR at level of femoral head.

Central Ray

- Utilizing hip localization method (p. 292), center CR to dependent femoral head.
- CR perpendicular to IR.

SID: 40 inches (100 cm)

Collimation Field

Size: Collimate on four sides to area of interest to include soft tissue margins.

Note: Dependent lower limb rotated 35 degrees medial (internally) in relationship to the IR.

Position

- The **superolateral aspect of acetabulum** with the femoral head centered within it.
- Proximal femoral head, neck and acetabulum is demonstrated

Exposure

- Optimal image receptor exposure and contrast; no motion
- Bony margins and sharp trabecular markings clearly seen

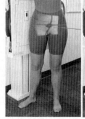 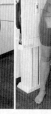

Fig. 5.34 AP oblique (false profile).

Fig. 5.35 AP oblique (modified profile).

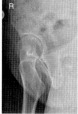 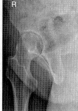

Fig. 5.36 *Left*, False Profile. *Right*, Modified False Profile. (From Atkins PR et al: Modified false-profile radiograph of the hip provides better visualization of the anterosuperior femoral head-neck junction. *Arthroscopy* 34(4):1236–1243.)

	cm	kVp	mA	Time	mAs	SID	Exposure Indicator
kVp Range:				75–85			
S							
M							
L							

Textbook, 11th ed, p. 289 and 290

AP and Lateral: Hips and Pelvis (Pediatric)

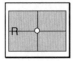

Warning: Do not attempt modified Cleaves hip position on trauma patients until fractures have been ruled out from the AP pelvis projection with possible hip pathology unless so indicated by a physician after review of the AP pelvis radiograph.

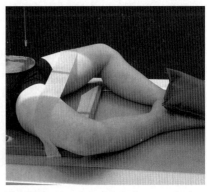

Fig. 5.37 Bilateral modified Cleaves method hips.

- IR size determined by size of body part to be radiographed; IR landscape
- Grid > 4 inches (10 cm)

Position (AP and Lateral)

- Patient should be supine, pelvis centered to CR and to IR; **use gonadal shields on both male and female** in accordance to local regulations, department policy and protocol. (Use ovarian shield of appropriate size for female, ensuring that it does not cover hip areas.)
- Immobilization techniques should be used when necessary to ensure pelvis is not rotated.

AP: Patient supine, extend legs, and internally rotate 15°

Frog-Leg Lateral

- Patient should be supine; flex knees and hips, place soles of feet together, knees bent and abducted. Bind soles of feet together, if needed.

Central Ray: CR ⊥, centered to level of hips

Minimum SID: 40 inches (100 cm)

Collimation Field Size: Collimate on four sides to area of interest to include soft tissue margins.

Respiration

- With infants and small children, watch their breathing pattern. When the abdomen is still, make the exposure.
- If the patient is crying, watch for the abdomen to be in full extension.

	cm	kVp	mA	Time	mAs	SID	Exposure Indicator
S							
M							
L							

Textbook, 11th ed, p. 647

5

Femur and Pelvis

Chapter 6

Vertebral Column

Intervertebral Foramina and Zygapophyseal Joints

Lateral and oblique projections best demonstrate these specific foramina and joints of the spine:

	Zygapophyseal Joints	Intervertebral Foramina
Cervical spine	Lateral position	45° anterior oblique (side closest to IR) 45° posterior oblique (side furthest to IR)
Thoracic spine	70° anterior oblique (side closest to IR)	Lateral position
Lumbar spine	45° posterior oblique (side closest to IR) 45° anterior oblique (side furthest to IR)	Lateral position

Topographic Landmarks

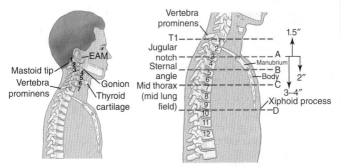

Fig. 6.1 Cervical spine landmarks.

Fig. 6.2 Sternum and thoracic spine landmarks.

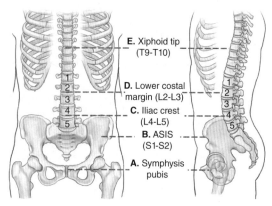

Fig. 6.3 Lower spine landmarks.

Digital Imaging Considerations

- **Four-sided collimation:** Collimate to the area of interest with a minimum of two (four is preferred) collimation parallel borders clearly demonstrated on the image.
- **Accurate centering:** The body part and the central ray (CR) should be centered to the IR.
- **Grid use with cassette-less systems:** Anatomy thickness and kVp range are deciding factors for whether a grid is to be used. With cassette-less systems, it may be impractical and difficult to remove the grid. Therefore, the grid is commonly left in place even for smaller body parts measuring < 4 inches (10 cm) or less. If grid is left in place, ensure the CR is centered to the grid. Virtual grid technology may eliminate the need for a physical grid.

AP "Open Mouth" C1–C2: Cervical Spine
Atlas and Axis

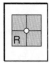

Warning: For trauma patients, do not remove cervical collar and do not move their head or neck until authorized by a physician who

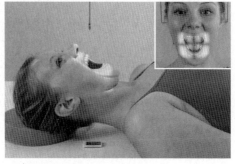

Fig. 6.4 AP open mouth for C1–C2.

has evaluated the horizontal beam lateral image or CT scan of the cervical spine.

- 8 × 10 inches (18 × 24 cm), portrait
- Grid
- AEC not recommended because of small field

Position

- Patient should be supine or erect and centered to CR and centerline.
- Adjust patient's head so that, with the mouth open, a plane from lower margin of upper incisors to the base of the skull (mastoid tips) is perpendicular to table or IR, or angle the CR accordingly.
- Center IR to CR.
- As a last step before making exposure, have patient open mouth wide without moving head (make final check for head alignment).

Central Ray: CR $\perp$ to IR through center of open mouth (to C1–C2)

SID: 40 inches (100 cm)

Collimation Field Size: Close collimation on four sides to C1–C2 region

Respiration: Suspend during exposure.

	cm	kVp	mA	Time	mAs	SID	Exposure Indicator
S							
M							
L							

kVp Range: 70–85

Textbook, 11th ed, 318

Vertebral Column

AP (PA) for Dens: Cervical Spine
AP (Fuchs Method) and PA (Judd Method)

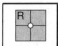

Warning: For trauma patients, do not remove cervical collar and do not move head or neck until authorized by a physician who has evaluated the horizontal beam lateral image or CT scan of the cervical spine. The cervical spine must be cleared for fracture or subluxation prior to performing these projections.

- 8 × 10 inches (18 × 24 cm), landscape
- Grid
- AEC not recommended

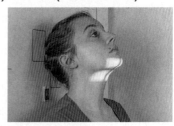

Fig. 6.5 AP Fuchs for dens (within foramen magnum outline).

Position

- Patient should be supine or erect, MSP aligned to centerline, no rotation.

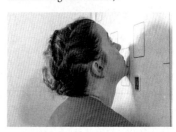

Fig. 6.6 PA Judd method.

- Elevate chin until MML is near ⊥ to IR (may require some cephalic CR angle if chin cannot be elevated sufficiently).

Note: The position may also be taken PA (Judd method) with chin against tabletop, using the same CR alignment.

- Center IR to exiting CR.

Central Ray: CR parallel to MML; 1 inch (2.5 cm) inferoposterior to mastoid tips and angles of mandible

SID: 40 inches (100 cm)

Collimation Field Size: Close collimation on all four sides to C1−C2 region

Respiration: Suspend during exposure.

kVp Range:					70–85		
	cm	kVp	mA	Time	mAs	SID	Exposure Indicator
S							
M							
L							

Textbook, 11th ed, p. 325

AP "Open Mouth" and AP (PA) Dens

Evaluation Criteria

Anatomy Demonstrated

- **Open mouth:** Dens (odontoid process) and vertebral body of C2, lateral masses and transverse processes of C1, and C1–C2 atlantoaxial joints
- **AP Fuchs:** Dens (odontoid process) within foramen magnum

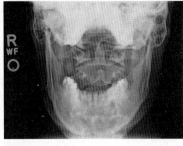

Fig. 6.7 AP open mouth—dens.

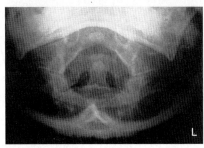

Fig. 6.8 AP (AP Fuchs—dens).

Position

- **Open mouth:** Upper incisors and base of the skull superimposed; entire dens demonstrated within foramen magnum
- **AP Fuchs:** Tip of mandible not superimposed over dens; symmetric appearance of mandible

Exposure

- Optimal image receptor exposure and contrast; no motion
- Soft tissue margins, bony margins, and trabecular markings; sharp outline of dens

AP Axial: Cervical Spine

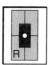

- 8 × 10 inches (18 × 24 cm) or 10 × 12 inches (24 × 30 cm), portrait
- Grid

Position

- Patient should be supine or erect; center midsagittal plane to CR (and to centerline of IR).
- Raise patient's chin slightly, as needed, so the CR angle superimposes the mentum of the mandible over the base of the skull (to prevent mandible from superimposing more than C1−C2).
- Center IR to projected CR.

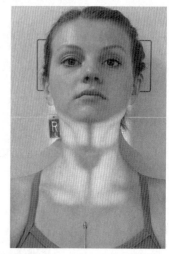

Fig. 6.9 Erect AP (CR 20° cephalad).

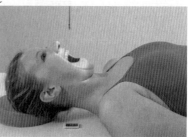

Fig. 6.10 Recumbent AP (CR 15° cephalad).

Central Ray: CR 15°−20° cephalad, to enter at C4 (inferior margin of thyroid cartilage)

SID: 40 inches (100 cm)

Collimation Field Size: Collimate on four sides to area of interest to include soft tissue margins

Respiration: Suspend during exposure.

	cm	kVp	mA	Time	mAs	SID	Exposure Indicator
S							
M							
L							

kVp Range: 70–85

Oblique: Cervical Spine

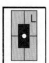

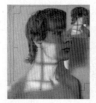

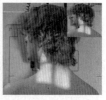

Warning: For trauma patients, do not remove cervical collar and do not move head or neck until authorized by a physician who

Fig. 6.11 LPO; CR 15° cephalad.

Fig. 6.12 RAO; CR 15° caudad.

has evaluated the horizontal beam lateral image or CT of the cervical spine.

Right and left obliques imaged for comparison (as either posterior or anterior obliques); **anterior obliques result in less thyroid dose**.

Skull rotation may vary between 45° and 90° from AP or PA position. Although the 45° degree may be ideal to demonstrate the intervertebral foramina without distortion, the mandible may obscure the region of C1 and C2. Follow department protocol on preferred degree of skull rotation:

- 10 × 12 inches (24 × 30 cm), portrait
- Grid (nongrid for cervical spine <10 cm thickness)

Position

- Patient should be erect (preferred), sitting or standing; rotate body 45° and skull into 45° (or 90°) oblique position, C spine aligned to CR (and centerline of IR).
- Have patient raise chin slightly, looking straight ahead (turn head slightly toward IR to prevent superimposing C1 by ramus of mandible).
- Center IR to projected CR.

Central Ray (Posterior Obliques): CR 15°–20° **cephalad**, to enter at C4; 15°–20° **caudad** angle required for anterior oblique

SID: 40–72 inches (100–180 cm); longer SID recommended

Collimation Field Size: Collimate on four sides to area of interest to include soft tissue margins

Respiration: Suspend during exposure.

	cm	kVp	mA	Time	mAs	SID	Exposure Indicator
S							
M							
L							

kVp Range: 70–85

Textbook, 11th ed, p. 320

AP Axial and Oblique: Cervical Spine

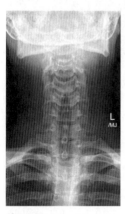 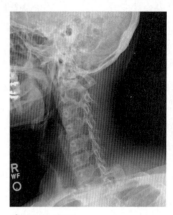

Fig. 6.13 AP axial.   **Fig. 6.14** RPO.

Evaluation Criteria

Anatomy Demonstrated

- **AP axial:** C3–T2 vertebral bodies and intervertebral joints
- **Oblique:** Intervertebral foramina open and pedicles
- **LPO/RPO projections:** Demonstrate upside (farthest from IR) intervertebral foramina and pedicles
- **LAO/RAO projections:** Demonstrate downside (closest to IR) intervertebral foramina and pedicles

Position

- **AP axial:** Intervertebral joints open and spinous processes equidistant to midline
- **Oblique:** 45° (AP or PA): Intervertebral foramina uniformly open and pedicles in profile

Exposure

- Optimal image receptor exposure and contrast; no motion
- Soft tissue and bony margins and trabecular markings sharp

Lateral (Erect): Cervical Spine

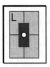

Trauma patients:
See Trauma Series:
Cervical Spine.

- 10 × 12 inches (24 × 30 cm), portrait
- Grid (nongrid for cervical spine <10 cm thickness)

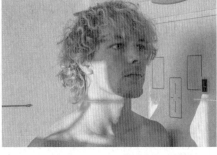

Fig. 6.15 Erect lateral, 72 inches (180 cm) SID.

Position

- Patient should be erect (sitting or standing) in lateral position, C spine aligned and centered to CR (and centerline of IR).
- Position top of IR ≈1–2 inches (2.5–5 cm) above level of EAM.
- Depress both shoulders evenly (weights in each hand may be necessary to visualize C7).
- Elevate patient's chin slightly (to remove mandible angles from spine).

Note: See the following page for swimmer's lateral if C7 is still not visualized.

Central Ray: CR $\perp$ IR horizontally to level of C4 (upper thyroid cartilage)

SID: 60–72 inches (150–180 cm) (Longer SID provides for better visualization of C7 because of less divergent rays.)

Collimation Field Size: Collimate on four sides to area of interest to include soft tissue margins

Respiration: Expose on full expiration.

	cm	kVp	mA	Time	mAs	SID	Exposure Indicator
S							
M							
L							

kVp Range: 70–85

Textbook, 11th ed, p. 321

6

Vertebral Column

Cervicothoracic (Swimmer's) Lateral: Cervical Spine

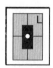

C5-T3 Region
- 10 × 12 inches (24 × 30 cm), portrait
- Grid

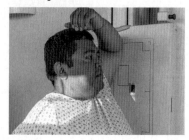

Fig. 6.16 Cervicothoracic (swimmer's) lateral.

Position
- Patient should be erect (preferred), sitting or standing; align C spine to CR (and centerline of IR).
- Place patient's arm and shoulder closest to the IR up, flexing elbow and resting forearm on head for support.
- Position arm and shoulder farthest from the IR down and rotate slightly posterior to place the remote humeral head posterior to vertebrae.
- Ensure that no rotation of thorax and head exists.

Central Ray: CR ⊥ centered to T1 (approximately 1 inch [2.5 cm] above level of jugular notch); **optional** 3°–5° caudad to separate the two shoulders for patient with limited flexibility

SID: 60–72 inches (150–180 cm)

Collimation Field Size: Collimate on four sides to area of interest to include soft tissue margins

Respiration: Expose on full expiration or orthostatic (breathing) technique.

kVp Range:				75–95			
	cm	kVp	mA	Time	mAs	SID	Exposure Indicator
S							
M							
L							

Textbook, 11th ed, p. 323

Lateral (Erect) and Cervicothoracic (Swimmer's) Lateral: Cervical Spine

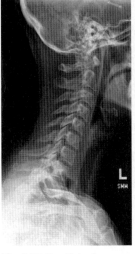 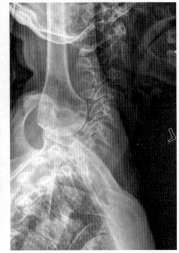

Fig. 6.17 Erect lateral.

Fig. 6.18 Cervicothoracic (swimmer's) lateral.

Evaluation Criteria

Anatomy Demonstrated

- **Lateral:** C1–C7 (minimum) intervertebral joint spaces and vertebral bodies demonstrated
- **Cervicothoracic:** Vertebral bodies and intervertebral disk spaces from C5–T3 (minimum) demonstrated

Position

- **Lateral:** Near superimposition of zygapophyseal joints; no superimposition of mandible on C spine
- **Cervicothoracic:** Separation of humeral heads from C spine; vertebral bodies in lateral perspective

Exposure

- Optimal image receptor exposure and contrast of lower cervical and upper thoracic spine; no motion
- Soft tissue margins and bony anatomy visible

6

Vertebral Column

Lateral (Hyperflexion and Hyperextension): Cervical Spine

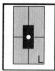

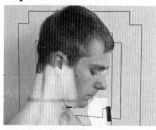

Fig. 6.19 Hyperflexion.

Warning: Functional study. Never attempt these positions on a trauma patient until authorized by a physician who has evaluated the horizontal beam lateral image or CT scan of the cervical spine.

- 10 × 12 inches (24 × 30 cm), portrait
- Grid (nongrid for cervical spine <10 cm thickness)

Position

- Patient should be erect (preferred) (sitting or standing)

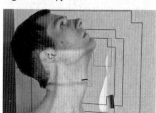

Fig. 6.20 Hyperextension.

in true lateral position, with no rotation of pelvis, shoulders, or head. C spine should be aligned to CR (and centerline of IR).
- Relax and depress shoulders as much as possible (weights on each arm may be used).

First IR: Hyperflexion: Depress chin to touch chest, if possible.
Second IR: Hyperextension: Elevate chin as far as is comfortable (entire C spine is included on both projections).
Central Ray: CR $\perp$ to C4 (level of upper margin of thyroid cartilage)
SID: 60–72 inches (150–180 cm)
Collimation Field Size: Collimate on four sides to area of interest to include soft tissue margins
Respiration: Expose on full expiration.

kVp Range:					70–85		
	cm	kVp	mA	Time	mAs	SID	Exposure Indicator
S							
M							
L							

Textbook, 11th ed, p. 324

Lateral (Hyperflexion and Hyperextension): Cervical Spine

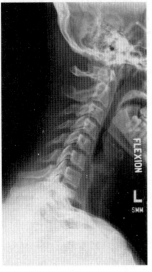

Fig. 6.21 Hyperflexion lateral.

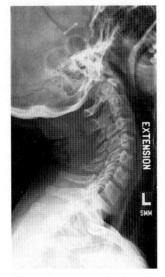

Fig. 6.22 Hyperextension lateral.

Evaluation Criteria

Anatomy Demonstrated
- **C1–C7:** Range of motion and ligament stability demonstrated

Position
- No rotation of head
- **Hyperflexion:** Spinous processes well separated
- **Hyperextension:** Spinous processes in close proximity

Exposure
- Optimal image receptor exposure and contrast; no motion
- Soft tissue margins visible and trabecular markings sharp

Trauma Series: Cervical Spine

Warning: For trauma patients, do not remove cervical collar and do not move head or neck until authorized by a physician who has evaluated the horizontal beam lateral image or CT of the cervical spine. Emergency departments routinely order CT to rule out fracture, subluxation, or other indications of cervical instability prior to performing any radiographic procedures.

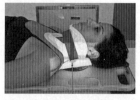

Fig. 6.23 Horizontal beam lateral.

Horizontal Beam Lateral
- 10 × 12 inches (24 × 30 cm), portrait
- Grid (nongrid for cervical spine <10 cm thickness)
- **SID:** 60–72 inches (150–180 cm)
- CR ⊥ to C4 (upper thyroid cartilage) (top of IR ≈1–2 inches or 3–5 cm above EAM)

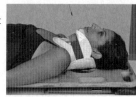

Fig. 6.24 AP axial.

AP
- Depress shoulders.
- 10 × 12 inches (24 × 30 cm), portrait
- Grid
- **SID:** 40–48 inches (100–120 cm)
- **CR:** 15°–20° cephalad, to enter at C4
- Expose upon full expiration.

AP Axial Oblique
- 10 × 12 inches (24 × 30 cm), portrait
- Grid
- **SID:** 40–48 inches (100–120 cm)
- **CR:** 45° medially (and 15° cephalad if nongrid)
- CR to enter at level of C4

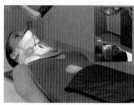

Fig. 6.25 Oblique (both R and L obliques).

Cervicothoracic Lateral
(Optional projection if needed to visualize C7)

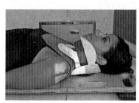

Fig. 6.26 Cervicothoracic lateral.

- 10 × 12 inches (24 × 30 cm), portrait
- Grid
- Elevate shoulder and arm nearest IR. Depress opposite shoulder.
- **SID:** 40–48 inches (100–120 cm)
- **CR:** IR centered to T1 (approximately 1.5 inches [2.5 cm] above level of jugular notch)

Textbook, 11th ed, p. 599

AP: Thoracic Spine

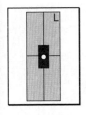

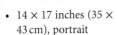

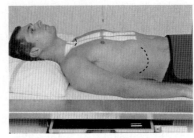

Fig. 6.27 AP thoracic spine.

- 14 × 17 inches (35 × 43 cm), portrait
- Grid
- Due to anode heel effect, it is necessary to place lower thoraco-lumbar spine at cathode end of x-ray tube.
- Compensating filter is useful in obtaining uniform brightness, density (thicker part of filter toward the upper vertebrae).

Position

- Patient supine, midsagittal plane aligned and centered to mid-line of table or IR; flex hips and knees to reduce lordotic curvature.
- Ensure top of IR is at least 1.5 inches (3 cm) above shoulder.
- Ensure no rotation of thorax or pelvis

Central Ray: CR ⊥ to center of IR (at level of T7 [as for an AP chest], 3–4 inches [8–10 cm] below jugular notch)

SID: 40 inches (100 cm)

Collimation Field Size: Collimate on four sides to area of interest to include soft tissue margins

Respiration: Expose on expiration for more uniform density.

	cm	kVp	mA	Time	mAs	SID	Exposure Indicator
kVp Range:					75–90		
S							
M							
L							

Textbook, 11th ed, p. 328

6

Vertebral Column

Lateral: Thoracic Spine

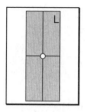

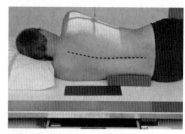

Fig. 6.28 Lateral thoracic spine.

- 14 × 17 inches (35 × 43 cm), portrait
- Grid
- Lead mat placed on table posterior to patient to reduce scatter to IR
- Do not use AEC if orthostatic breathing technique is used.

Position

- Patient should be recumbent, support under head, lateral with knees flexed, arms raised, and elbows flexed.
- Align and center midaxillary plane to midline of table or IR.
- Ensure top of IR is at least 1.5 inches (3 cm) above shoulders; no rotation.
- Supports should be placed under lower back, as needed, to straighten and align spine near parallel to tabletop.

Central Ray: CR $\perp$ to center of IR T7 (3–4 inches [8–10 cm] below jugular notch or 7–8 inches [18–20 cm] below the vertebra prominens). A patient with broad shoulders may require a 10°–15° cephalic CR angle if waist is not supported.

SID: 40 inches (100 cm)

Collimation Field Size: Collimate on four sides to area of interest to include soft tissue margins

Respiration: Orthostatic (breathing) technique is recommended—minimum of 2–3 seconds; or expose on full inspiration.

	cm	kVp	mA	Time	mAs	SID	Exposure Indicator
S							
M							
L							

kVp Range: 80–95

Textbook, 11th ed, p. 329

AP and Lateral: Thoracic Spine

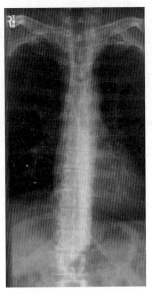

Fig. 6.29 AP thoracic spine.

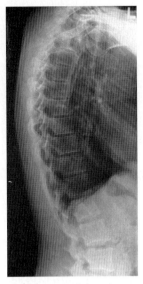

Fig. 6.30 Lateral thoracic spine (suspended respiration).

Evaluation Criteria

Anatomy Demonstrated
- **AP and lateral:** 12 thoracic bodies, intervertebral joint spaces, and spinous and transverse processes

Position
- **AP:** SC joints equidistant from midline, no rotation
- **Lateral:** Intervertebral disk spaces open

Exposure
- Optimal image receptor exposure and contrast; no motion on AP projection. Orthostatic (breathing) technique for lateral projection is desirable.
- Soft tissue should be margins visible and trabecular markings sharp.

Oblique: Thoracic Spine

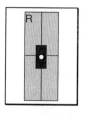

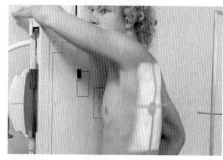

Fig. 6.31 70° RAO (20° from lateral).

Both oblique projections are generally imaged for comparison. Anterior oblique is recommended (lower breast dose).

- 14 × 17 inches (35 × 43 cm), portrait
- Grid

Position

- Patient should be recumbent or erect, rotated anteriorly 20° from true lateral to create a **70° oblique** from plane of table.
- Align and center spine to midline of table /or IR; place arm nearest from IR down and posterior; arm closest to tube up in front of head.
- Ensure top of IR is at least 1.5 inches (3 cm) above shoulders.

Central Ray: CR ⊥ to center of IR to T7 (7–8 inches [18–20 cm] below vertebra prominens or 2 inches [5 cm] below sternal angle)

SID: 40 inches (100 cm)

Collimation Field Size: Collimate on four sides to area of interest to include soft tissue margins

Respiration: Expose on expiration.

kVp Range:					80–95		
	cm	kVp	mA	Time	mAs	SID	Exposure Indicator
S							
M							
L							

Textbook, 11th ed, p. 330

AP (PA): Lumbar Spine

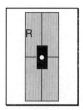

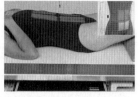

Fig. 6.32 AP lumbar (recumbent and erect).

Note: May be performed PA, which places intervertebral spaces more closely parallel to the diverging rays.

- 14 × 17 inches (35 × 43 cm), portrait
- Grid

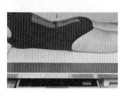

Fig. 6.33 Alternate PA.

Position (AP)

- Patient should be supine or erect, midsagittal plane aligned to midline of table or grid.
- Flex hips and knees (to reduce lordotic curvature) for recumbent position.
- No rotation of thorax or pelvis needed (ASISs should be same distance from table).
- Center IR to CR.

Central Ray

- CR ⊥ to IR
- More open collimation: 14 × 17 inches (35 × 43 cm). Direct CR to **level of iliac crest** (L4–L5). This larger IR will include lumbar vertebrae, sacrum, and possibly coccyx.
- Tighter collimation: Direct CR to level of L3, which may be localized by palpation of the lower costal margin (1.5 inches [4 cm] above iliac crest). This tighter collimation will include primarily the five lumbar vertebrae.

SID: 40 inches (100 cm)

Collimation Field Size: Collimate on four sides to area of interest to include soft tissue margins

Respiration: Expose at end of expiration.

	cm	kVp	mA	Time	mAs	SID	Exposure Indicator
S							
M							
L							

kVp Range: 75–90

Textbook, 11th ed, p. 345

AP (PA): Lumbar Spine

Evaluation Criteria

Anatomy Demonstrated

- Lumbar vertebral bodies, inter-vertebral joints, spinous and transverse processes, SI joints, and sacrum
- More open collimation: approximately T11 to the distal sacrum
- Tighter collimation: T12 to S1 included

Position

- No rotation is evident by symmetry of transverse processes, SI joints, and sacrum.
- Spinous processes are midline.
- Open intervertebral joint spaces.

Exposure

- Optimal image receptor exposure and contrast; no motion
- Soft tissue margins and sharp trabecular markings clearly demonstrated

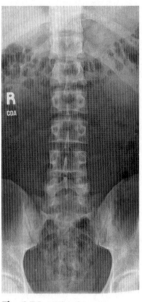

Fig. 6.34 AP lumbar spine.

Oblique: Lumbar Spine

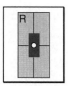

Both oblique projections are performed for comparison (as either anterior or posterior obliques).

- 10 × 12 inches (24 × 30 cm), portrait
- Grid

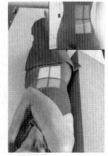

Fig. 6.35 Posterior oblique-recumbent (45° LPO) and erect (45° RPO).

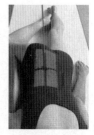

Fig. 6.36 Anterior oblique (45° LAO).

Position

- Patient should be recumbent or erect, rotate body 45° and right and left posterior or anterior obliques (use support angle blocks under pelvis and shoulders to maintain position for recumbent posterior obliques).
- Align and center spine to CR and midline of table or IR.

Central Ray: CR ⊥ to body of L3 at level of lower costal margin (1–2 inches [2.5–5 cm] above iliac crest) and 2 inches (5 cm) medial to upside ASIS

SID: 40 inches (100 cm)

Collimation Field Size: Collimate on four sides to area of interest to include soft tissue margins

Respiration: Suspend during exposure

Note: 50° oblique is best for L1–L2 zygapophyseal joints.

	cm	kVp	mA	Time	mAs	SID	Exposure Indicator
S							
M							
L							

kVp Range: 75–90

Textbook, 11th ed, p. 346

Oblique: Lumbar Spine

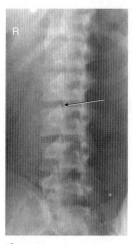
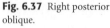

Fig. 6.37 Right posterior oblique.

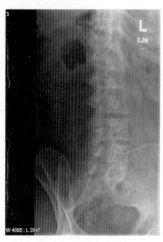

Fig. 6.38 Left posterior oblique.

Evaluation Criteria

Anatomy Demonstrated

- **LPO/RPO:** L1–L4 downside zygapophyseal joints. Scottie dog elements are visible.
- **LAO/RAO:** L1–L4 upside zygapophyseal joints. Scottie dog elements are visible.

Position

- Zygapophyseal joints and pedicle ("eye") centered on the vertebral body

Exposure

- Optimal image receptor exposure and contrast; no motion
- Soft tissue margins visible and bony detail of vertebral bodies, joint spaces, and elements of Scottie dog (arrows indicate zygapophyseal joints)

Lateral: Lumbar Spine

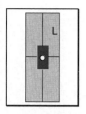

Fig. 6.39 Lateral L spine (recumbent and erect).

- 14 × 17 inches (35 × 43 cm), portrait
- Grid
- Due to anode heel effect, place lumbar spine at cathode end of x-ray tube.
- Lead masking should be posterior to patient.

Position
- Patient should be recumbent or erect in true lateral position; flex hips and knees, align and center midaxillary plane to centerline.
- Place support under the waist, as needed, to place entire spine parallel to tabletop (see **Note**). Provide support between knees for recumbent position.
- Center IR to CR.

Central Ray
- CR perpendicular to IR
- More open collimation: Center to level of iliac crest (L4–L5). This projection includes lumbar vertebrae, sacrum, and possibly coccyx.
- Tighter collimation: Center to L3 at the level of the lower costal margin (1.5 inches [4 cm] above iliac crest). This includes the five lumbar vertebrae.

SID: 40 inches (100 cm)

Collimation Field Size: Collimate on four sides to area of interest to include soft tissue margins

Respiration: Expose at end of expiration.

Note: Patient with wide pelvis and narrow thorax may require a 3°–5° caudal CR angle, even with support under waist. If patient has natural lateral curvature (scoliosis), place "sag" or convexity down.

kVp Range:				80–90			
	cm	kVp	mA	Time	mAs	SID	Exposure Indicator
S							
M							
L							

Textbook, 11th ed, p. 347

6

Vertebral Column

Lateral L5–S1: Lumbar Spine

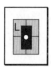

- 8 × 10 inches (18 × 24 cm), portrait
- Grid
- Lead masking posterior to patient

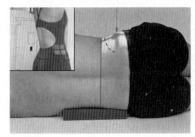

Fig. 6.40 Lateral L5–S1 (recumbent and erect).

Position
- Patient should be erect or recumbent in true lateral position; flex hips and knees, midaxillary plane aligned to midline of table or IR and CR.
- Place support under waist, as needed for recumbent position, to place entire spine parallel to tabletop. Provide support between knees.
- Center IR to CR.

Central Ray
- CR ⊥ to IR if entire spine is parallel to table; or 5°–8° caudad if entire spine is not parallel (most often on females); angle CR to be parallel to the **interiliac plane**
- CR to 1.5 inches (4 cm) inferior to iliac crest and 2 inches (5 cm) posterior to ASIS
- Center IR to CR.

SID: 40 inches (100 cm)

Collimation Field Size: Collimate on four sides to area of interest to include soft tissue margins

Respiration: Suspend during exposure.

	cm	kVp	mA	Time	mAs	SID	Exposure Indicator
S							
M							
L							

kVp Range: 85–95

Textbook, 11th ed, p. 349

6

Vertebral Column

Lateral and Lateral L5–S1: Lumbar Spine

Evaluation Criteria

Anatomy Demonstrated
- **Lateral:** L1–L4 vertebral bodies, intervertebral joints, and foramina and spinous processes
- **Lateral L5–S1:** Open L5–S1 vertebral bodies, intervertebral joint spaces, and intervertebral foramina

Position
- **Lateral:** Vertebral column parallel to IR; intervertebral joint spaces and foramina open; no rotation
- **Lateral L5–S1:** Intervertebral joint spaces and intervertebral foramina open; no rotation

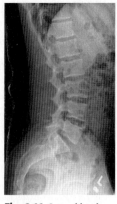

Fig. 6.41 Lateral lumbar spine.

Exposure
- Optimal image receptor exposure and contrast; no motion
- Soft tissue margins visible and bony detail of vertebral bodies, joint spaces, and spinous process

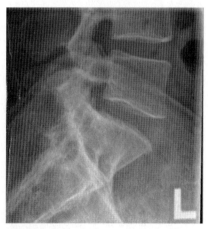

Fig. 6.42 Lateral L5–S1.

PA: Scoliosis Series
Ferguson Method

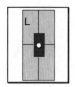

PA greatly reduces dose to radiation-sensitive areas and is strongly recommended over AP projection. Radiologic technologists should follow local regulations, department policy and protocol in the use of breast and gonadal shielding.

A scoliosis series may include two PA projections: one standard erect PA and one with the foot or hip on the **convex side** of the curve elevated

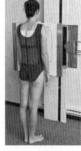

Fig. 6.43 PA without block.

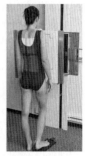

Fig. 6.44 PA with block under foot on convex side of curve.

- 14 × 17 inches (35 × 43 cm), portrait, or 14 × 36 inches (35 × 90 cm), portrait
- Grid
- Compensating filters to obtain a more uniform density along the vertebral column

Position
First Image
- Patient should be erect, standing or seated, spine aligned and centered to midline of table or IR, arms at side, no rotation of pelvis or thorax.
- Distribute weight evenly on both feet for the erect position.
- Lower margin of IR 1–2 inches (2.5–5 cm) below iliac crest.

Second Image: Place 3- to 4-inch (8- to 10-cm) block under foot (or buttock if seated) on **convex side** of curvature so that the patient can barely maintain position **without assistance**.

Central Ray: CR ⊥ to center of IR

SID: 40–60 inches (100–150 cm); longer SID is recommended

Collimation Field Size: Collimate on four sides to area of interest to include soft tissue margins

Respiration: On full expiration.

kVp Range:						75–90	
	cm	kVp	mA	Time	mAs	SID	Exposure Indicator
S							
M							
L							

AP: Lumbar Spine
Right and Left Bending

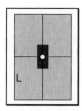

Note: May be taken erect PA to reduce dose to radiation-sensitive areas.

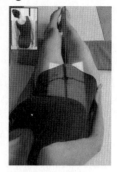

Fig. 6.45 AP, right bending-recumbent and erect

Fig. 6.46 AP, left bending-recumbent and erect

- 14 × 17 inches (35 × 43 cm), portrait, or 14 × 36 inches (35 × 90 cm), portrait
- Grid
- Compensating filters to produce a more uniform density of spine

Position

- Patient should be erect (preferred) or recumbent, midsagittal plane centered to CR and midline of table or IR.
- Bend laterally as far as possible (right then left) without tilting pelvis (pelvis remains stationary and acts as a fulcrum).
- Ensure no rotation of thorax or pelvis.
- Lower margin of IR 1–2 inches (2.5–5 cm) below iliac crest.

Central Ray: CR $\perp$ to center of IR (higher centering if thoracic spine is area of interest)

SID: 40–60 inches (100–150 cm)

Collimation Field Size: Collimate on four sides to area of interest to include soft tissue margins

Respiration: Expose at end of expiration.

	cm	kVp	mA	Time	mAs	SID	Exposure Indicator
S							
M							
L							

kVp Range: 80–95

Textbook, 11th ed, p. 355

6

Vertebral Column

Lateral (Hyperflexion and Hyperextension): Lumbar Spine

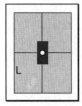

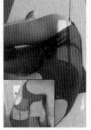

Fig. 6.47
Hyperflexion
lateral-recumbent
and erect.

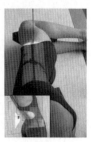

Fig. 6.48
Hyperextension
lateral-recumbent
and erect.

Two images are obtained with the patient in the lateral position (one in hyperflexion and one in hyperextension):

- 14 × 17 inches (35 × 43 cm), portrait
- Grid
- Lead masking posterior to patient

Position

- Patient should be erect (preferred) or recumbent, midcoronal plane centered to table
- Support under waist to align spine parallel to tabletop.
- Hyperflex forward as far as possible, then hyperextend back as far as possible for second IR; maintain true lateral position.
- Lower margin of IR 1–2 inches (2.5–5 cm) below iliac crest.

Central Ray: CR ⊥ to center of IR (or to site of fusion if known)
SID: 40 inches (100 cm)
Collimation Field Size: Collimate on four sides to area of interest to include soft tissue margins
Respiration: Expose at end of expiration.

	cm	kVp	mA	Time	mAs	SID	Exposure Indicator
kVp Range:					80–95		
S							
M							
L							

Textbook, 11th ed, p. 356

Lateral (Hyperflexion and Hyperextension): Lumbar Spine

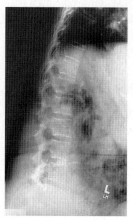

Fig. 6.49 Hyperflexion lateral.

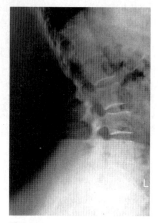

Fig. 6.50 Hyperextension lateral.

Evaluation Criteria

Anatomy Demonstrated

- **Hyperflexion:** Thoracic and lumbar vertebra including 1–2 inches (≈3–5 cm) of the iliac crests; lateral view of lumbar vertebrae in hyperflexion
- **Hyperextension:** Thoracic and lumbar vertebra including 1–2 inches (≈3–5 cm) of the iliac crests; lateral view of lumbar vertebrae in hyperextension

Position

- **Hyperflexion:** True lateral with no rotation; spaces between spinous processes open
- **Hyperextension:** True lateral with no rotation; spaces between spinous processes closed

Exposure

- Optimal image receptor exposure and contrast; no motion
- Bony detail of vertebral bodies, spinous processes, and intervertebral joint spaces

6

Vertebral Column

AP Axial: Sacrum

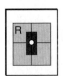

- 10 × 12 inches (24 × 30 cm), portrait
- Grid

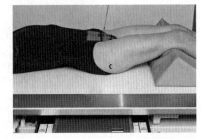

Fig. 6.51 AP sacrum, CR 15° cephalad.

Position
- Patient supine, midsagittal plane centered to CR and midline of table or IR
- No rotation of pelvis needed (both ASIS same distance from table)
- Center IR to projected CR

Central Ray: CR 15° cephalad, at 2 inches (5 cm) superior to pubic symphysis

SID: 40 inches (100 cm)

Collimation Field Size: Collimate on four sides to area of interest to include soft tissue margins

Respiration: Suspend during exposure.

	cm	kVp	mA	Time	mAs	SID	Exposure Indicator
S							
M							
L							

kVp Range: 75–90

Textbook, 11th ed, p. 358

AP Axial: Coccyx

Note: May be performed PA with a 10° cephalic angle if the patient cannot sustain weight on the coccyx area in a supine position. Position may be performed erect.

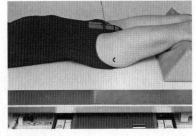

Fig. 6.52 AP axial coccyx, CR 10° caudad.

Urinary bladder should be emptied before procedure is performed.

- 8 × 10 inches (18 × 24 cm), portrait
- Grid
  AEC is discouraged

Position

- Patient should be supineand support under knees
- Align and center midsagittal plane to midline of table or IR, no rotation.
- Center IR to level of projected CR.

Central Ray: CR 10° caudad, centered to 2 inches (5 cm) superior to symphysis pubis

SID: 40 inches (100 cm)

Collimation Field Size: Collimate on four sides to area of interest to include soft tissue margins

Respiration: Suspend during exposure.

	cm	kVp	mA	Time	mAs	SID	Exposure Indicator
S							
M							
L							

kVp Range: 75–85

Textbook, 11th ed, p. 359

AP Axial: Sacrum and Coccyx

Evaluation Criteria

Anatomy Demonstrated

- **AP sacrum:** Nonforeshortened image of sacrum
- **AP coccyx:** Nonforeshortened image of coccyx

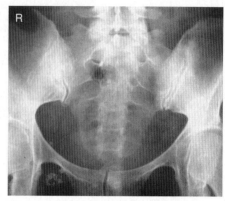

Fig. 6.53 AP axial sacrum.

Position

- **AP sacrum:** Sacrum free of superimposition and sacral foramina visible
- **AP coccyx:** Coccyx free of superimposition and not rotated

Exposure

- Optimal image receptor exposure and contrast; no motion
- Soft tissue visible and sharp bony detail

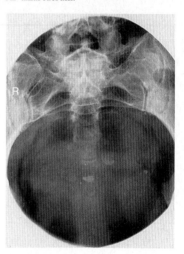

Fig. 6.54 AP axial coccyx.

Lateral: Sacrum and Coccyx

Note: Lateral sacrum and lateral coccyx may be performed as one projection if both sacrum and coccyx are being examined (reduces patient exposure). Position may be performed erect.

- 10 × 12 inches (24 × 30 cm), portrait
- Grid
- Lead masking posterior to patient
- If coccyx is to be included, a compensating (boomerang-type) filter is useful to ensure optimal density.

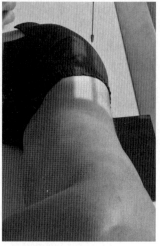

Fig. 6.55 Lateral sacrum and coccyx.

Position

- Patient lateral recumbent, hips and knees flexed, true lateral position
- Center sacrum to CR and midline of table or IR (Align patient and IR to correctly centered CR.).

Central Ray (Sacrum): CR ⊥, directed to 3–4 inches (8–10 cm) posterior to upside ASIS

SID: 40 inches (100 cm)

Collimation Field Size: Collimate on four sides to area of interest to include soft tissue margins

Respiration: Suspend during exposure.

	cm	kVp	mA	Time	mAs	SID	Exposure Indicator
kVp Range:					85–95		
S							
M							
L							

Textbook, 11th ed, p. 360

Lateral: Sacrum and Coccyx

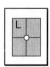

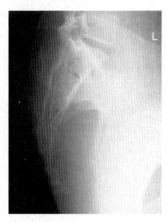

Fig. 6.56 Lateral sacrum and coccyx.

Evaluation Criteria
Anatomy Demonstrated
- Lateral view of sacrum and coccyx
- Lateral view of L5–S1 inter-vertebral joint

Position
- No rotation evident by greater sciatic notches, and femoral heads superimposed
- Entire sacrum and coccyx included

Exposure
- Optimal image receptor exposure and contrast; no motion
- Trabecular markings clearly demonstrated

AP Axial: Sacroiliac (SI) Joint

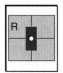

- 10 × 12 inches (24 × 30 cm), portrait
- Grid

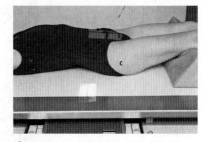

Fig. 6.57 AP axial SI joints (CR 30°–35° cephalad).

Position

- Patient should be supine; align midsagittal plane to midline of table or IR.
- No rotation of pelvis needed (ASISs the same distance from tabletop).
- Center IR to projected CR.

Central Ray: CR 30° (males) and 35° (females) cephalad, 2 inches (5 cm) below level of ASIS

SID: 40 inches (100 cm)

Collimation Field Size: Collimate on four sides to area of interest to include soft tissue margins

Respiration: Suspend during exposure.

kVp Range:					80–95		
	cm	kVp	mA	Time	mAs	SID	Exposure Indicator
S							
M							
L							

Textbook, 11th ed, p. 361

Posterior Oblique: Sacroiliac (SI) Joint

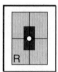

- 10 × 12 inches (24 × 30 cm), portrait
- Grid
- Bilateral study for comparison
- May be performed erect

Position

- Patient should be supine in 25°–30° posterior oblique with side of interest elevated (use support to maintain this position).

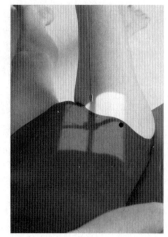

Fig. 6.58 25°–30° LPO for upside (right) SI joint.

- Align elevated SI joint to CR and to midline of table or IR (1 inch [2.5 cm] medial to upside ASIS).
- Center IR to CR.

Central Ray: CR ⊥ to 1 inch (2.5 cm) medial to upside ASIS

SID: 40 inches (100 cm)

Collimation Field Size: Collimate on four sides to area of interest to include soft tissue margins

Respiration: Suspend during exposure.

Note: CR may be angled 15°–20° cephalad to best demonstrate the distal part of joint

	cm	kVp	mA	Time	mAs	SID	Exposure Indicator
S							
M							
L							

kVp Range: 80–95

Textbook, 11th ed, p. 362

Posterior Oblique: Sacroiliac Joint

Evaluation Criteria
Anatomy Demonstrated
- Open upside (farthest from IR) SI joint

Position
- **LPO:** Right SI joint open; no overlap of iliac wing and sacrum
- **RPO:** Left SI joint open; no overlap of iliac wing and sacrum

Exposure
- Optimal image receptor exposure and contrast; no motion
- Bony margins and sharp trabecular markings clearly demonstrated

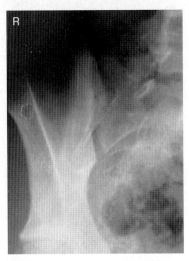

Fig. 6.59 LPO projection of (right) SI joint.

Vertebral Column

Chapter 7

Bony Thorax

(R) Routine, (S) Special

Positioning Considerations
Sternum

The routine examination for a sternum generally includes a lateral and an oblique wherein the sternum is shifted to the left of the spine and is superimposed over the homogeneous heart shadow. A 15°–20° RAO achieves this best. An orthostatic-breathing technique is typically used to blur out the lung markings and the ribs overlying the sternum. If preferred, exposure can also be made on suspended expiration. A minimum SID for sternum imaging is 40 inches (100 cm). To minimize the dose, the patient's skin should be at least 15 inches (38 cm) below the surface of the collimator.

Ribs

Specific projections performed in a radiographic examination of the ribs are determined by the patient's clinical history and department protocol. If the referring physician does not provide the patient's history, the technologist must obtain a complete clinical history.

Two-Image Routine

A suggested two-image routine is an **AP** or **PA** with the area of interest closest to the image receptor (IR) (above or below diaphragm) and an **oblique** projection of the axillary ribs on the side of the injury. Therefore, the oblique for this routine on an injury to the left anterior ribs would be an RAO, shifting the spine away from the area of injury and increasing the visibility of the left axillary ribs. The oblique for an injury to the right posterior ribs would be an RPO wherein the spine again is rotated away from the area of injury. Note that certain departments require the right and left thorax be demonstrated on the oblique projections.

Three-Image Routine

A three-image routine is required in some departments for all rib trauma consisting of **AP above diaphragm** or **AP below diaphragm** and **RPO** and **LPO** of the site of injury.

Above and Below Diaphragm

The location of the injury site in relationship to the diaphragm is important for all routines. Injuries above the diaphragm require less exposure (nearer to a chest technique) when taken on **inspiration**, and those below the diaphragm require an exposure nearer to that of an abdomen technique when taken on **expiration**.

Right Anterior Oblique (RAO): Sternum

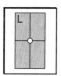

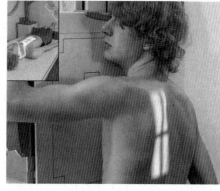

Fig. 7.1 Erect 15°–20° RAO sternum (*inset:* trauma option).

- 10 × 12 inches (24 × 30 cm), portrait
- Grid
- Orthostatic-breathing technique (2–3 seconds)* or suspended expiration
- AEC not recommended

Position

- Patient erect (preferred) or semiprone, body turned 15°–20° with right side down (RAO) (A hyposthenic patient requires slightly more obliquity than a hypersthenic patient.)
- Center sternum to CR at midline of table or IR holder

Central Ray: CR ⊥ to center of sternum (1 inch [2.5 cm] to left of midline and midway between jugular notch and xiphoid process)

SID: 40 inches (100 cm)

Collimation Field Size: Collimate on four sides to area of interest to include soft tissue margins

*Orthostatic technique is not recommended for the erect RAO position. The thorax tends to move even during quiet respiration.

	cm	kVp	mA	Time	mAs	SID	Exposure Indicator
S							
M							
L							

kVp Range: 70–85

Textbook, 11th ed, p. 374

Lateral: Sternum

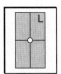

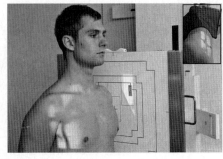

- 10 × 12 inches (24 × 30 cm), portrait, or 14 × 17 inches (35 × 35 cm), portrait

Fig. 7.2 Lateral, erect sternum (*inset:* trauma option).

- Grid
- AEC not recommended
- Place lead blocker anterior to sternum (for recumbent position).

Position

- Patient erect (preferred) (seated or standing), or lateral recumbent lying on side with vertical CR, or supine with cross-table CR for severe trauma
- Arms up above head and shoulders back
- Sternum aligned to CR at midline of grid or table/upright bucky
- Top of IR 1.5 inches (4 cm) above the jugular notch

Central Ray: CR ⊥ to center of sternum

SID: 60–72 inches (150–180 cm) recommended, 40 inches (100 cm) minimum

Collimation Field Size: Collimate on four sides to area of interest to include soft tissue margins

Respiration: Expose upon **full inspiration**.

	cm	kVp	mA	Time	mAs	SID	Exposure Indicator
kVp Range:				75–85			
S							
M							
L							

Textbook, 11ᵗʰ ed, p. 375

Bony Thorax

7

227

Oblique (RAO): Sternum

Evaluation Criteria

Anatomy Demonstrated

- Entire sternum superimposed on heart shadow

Position

- Correct patient rotation, sternum visualized alongside vertebral column

Exposure

- Optimal image receptor exposure and contrast to visualize entire sternum
- A 2- to 3-second exposure using breathing technique; lung markings appear blurred
- Bony margins sharp

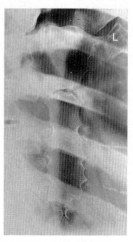

Fig. 7.3 RAO sternum.

Lateral: Sternum

Evaluation Criteria

Anatomy Demonstrated

- Entire sternum with minimal overlap of soft tissues

Position

- No rotation, sternum visualized with no superimposition on the ribs
- Shoulders and arms drawn back

Exposure

- Optimal contrast and density (brightness); no motion
- Sharp bony margins

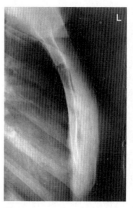

Fig. 7.4 Lateral sternum.

PA and Anterior Oblique: Sternoclavicular (SC) Joints

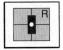

- 8 × 10 inches (18 × 24 cm), landscape
- Grid

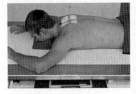

Fig. 7.5 Bilateral PA.

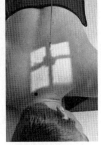

Fig. 7.6 RAO, 10°–15° oblique, CR ⊥ (both obliques commonly taken for comparison).

Position

PA: Patient prone or erect, midsagittal plane to centerline of CR
- Turn head to side, no rotation of shoulders.
- Center **IR** to **CR**.

Oblique: Rotate thorax 10°–15° to shift vertebrae away from sternum (best visualizes **downside** SC joint). **RAO** will demonstrate the right SC joint. **LAO** will demonstrate the left SC joint. Less obliquity (5°–10°) will best visualize the upside SC joint next to spine.

Central Ray
- **PA:** Level of T2–T3; CR ⊥ to MSP and ≈3 inches (7 cm) distal to vertebra prominens (spinous process of C7)
- **Oblique:** Level of T2–T3; CR ⊥ to 1–2 inches (2.5–5 cm) lateral to MSP (toward elevated side) and ≈3 inches (7 cm) distal to vertebra prominens

SID: 40 inches (100 cm)

Collimation Field Size: Collimate on four sides to area of interest to include soft tissue margins

Respiration: Suspend upon expiration.

Bony Thorax

7

kVp Range:					75–85	
	cm	kVp	mA	Time	mAs	SID	Exposure Indicator
S							
M							
L							

Textbook, 11ᵗʰ ed, pp. 376 and 377

PA: SC Joints

Evaluation Criteria
Anatomy Demonstrated
- Bilateral right and left sternoclavicular joints. Lateral aspect of manubrium and medial portion of clavicles visualized lateral to vertebral column.

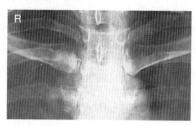

Fig. 7.7 PA bilateral SC joints.

Position
- No rotation, equal distance of SC joints from vertebral column

Exposure
- Optimal image receptor exposure and contrast to visualize SC joints; no motion
- SC joints visualized through ribs and lungs
- Sharp bony margins

Anterior Oblique: SC Joints

Evaluation Criteria
Anatomy Demonstrated
- Manubrium and medial clavicles and downside SC joints are visualized.

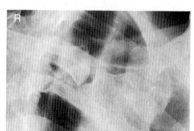

Fig. 7.8 10°–15° RAO.

Position
- Patient rotated 10°–15°; correct rotation best demonstrates downside SC joint with no superimposition of vertebral column

Exposure
- Contrast and density (brightness) sufficient to visualize SC joint through ribs and lungs; no motion
- Sharp bony margins

AP (or PA): Ribs (Bilateral)
Above Diaphragm

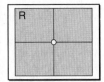

Generally taken as AP for posterior ribs and PA for anterior ribs:

- 14 × 17 inches (35 × 43 cm), landscape (or portrait for unilateral study or narrow chest dimensions)
- Grid

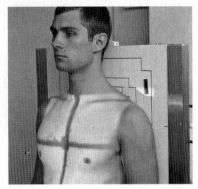

Fig. 7.9 AP bilateral ribs above diaphragm.

Position
- Patient should be erect (preferred), or recumbent, midsagittal plane to midline of table/upright bucky and CR.
- Position top of IR ≈1.5 inches (4 cm) above shoulders.
- Roll shoulders forward, no rotation.
- Ensure that thorax is centered to IR (bilateral study).

Central Ray: CR ⊥ IR, centered to the midsagittal plane, at a level 3 or 4 inches (8–10 cm) below jugular notch (level of T7)

SID: 72 inches (180 cm) erect; 40–48 inches (100–120 cm) recumbent

Collimation Field Size: Collimate on four sides to area of interest to include soft tissue margins

Respiration: Expose on **inspiration** (diaphragm down).

	cm	kVp	mA	Time	mAs	SID	Exposure Indicator
kVp Range:				75–85			
S							
M							
L							

Textbook, 11th ed, p. 378

AP: Ribs (Bilateral)
Below Diaphragm

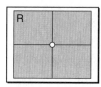

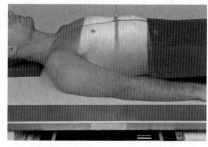

Fig. 7.10 AP bilateral ribs below diaphragm.

- 14 × 17 inches (35 × 43 cm), landscape (or portrait for unilateral study or narrow chest dimensions)
- Grid

Position

- Patient should be erect, or recumbent, MSP to midline of table/upright bucky and IR (and CR).
- Raise chin to prevent superimposition of upper ribs.
- Rotate shoulders anteriorly to remove scapulae from lung fields.

Note: Some routines include only unilateral ribs of affected side.

Central Ray: CR ⊥ to IR, centered to the midsagittal plane at a level midway between the xiphoid process and the lower rib margin

SID: 72 inches (180 cm) erect; 40 inches (100 cm) recumbent

Collimation Field Size: Collimate on four sides to area of interest to include soft tissue margins

Respiration: Expose on **expiration** (diaphragm at highest point).

	cm	kVp	mA	Time	mAs	SID	Exposure Indicator
kVp Range:					75–85		
S							
M							
L							

Textbook, 11th ed, p. 378

AP (or PA): Ribs (Bilateral)
Above and Below Diaphragm

Evaluation Criteria

Anatomy Demonstrated:

Above Diaphragm
- Ribs 1–9 visualized

Below Diaphragm
- Ribs 10–12 (minimum) visualized

Position
- No rotation, lateral rib margins equal distance from vertebral column

Exposure
- Optimal image receptor exposure and contrast appropriate to visualize ribs 1–10 above diaphragm and 10–12 (minimum) below diaphragm; no motion
- Sharp bony margins

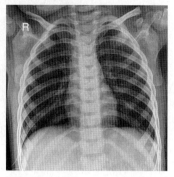

Fig. 7.11 PA bilateral ribs above diaphragm.

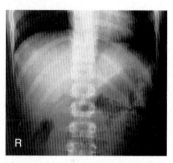

Fig. 7.12 AP bilateral ribs below diaphragm.

Anterior Oblique (RAO): Upper Axillary Ribs

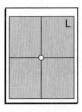

- 14 × 17 inches (35 × 43), or 14 × 14 inches (35 × 35 cm), landscape (see **Note**)
- Grid

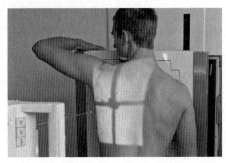

Fig. 7.13 A 45° RAO above diaphragm—for left anterior and axillary rib injury.

Position

- Patient should be erect (preferred) or recumbent if needed.
- Oblique 45° (affected side away from IR), rotate spine away from area of interest.
- Abduct downside arm away from thorax; elevate opposite arm away from thorax.
- Align a plane of the thorax midway between the spine and the lateral margin of thorax on side of interest to CR and to midline of the grid or table/bucky.

Note: Some routines indicate unilateral oblique only of the affected side with a smaller IR placed portrait.

Central Ray: CR ⊥ to IR, centered to level 7–8 inches (18–20 cm) below vertebra prominens (T7)

SID: 72 inches (180 cm) erect, 40 inches (100 cm) recumbent

Collimation Field Size: Collimate on four sides to area of interest to include soft tissue margins

Respiration: Above diaphragm—expose on **inspiration**.

	cm	kVp	mA	Time	mAs	SID	Exposure Indicator
kVp Range:					75–85		
S							
M							
L							

Textbook, 11th ed, p. 382

Posterior Oblique (LPO): Lower Axillary Ribs

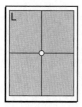

- 14 × 17 inches (35 × 43 cm), or 14 × 14 inches (35 × 35), portrait
- Grid

Position

- Patient should be erect (preferred) or recumbent if needed.
- Oblique 45° (affected side away from IR); rotate spine away from area of interest.

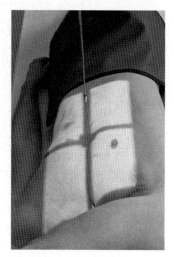

Fig. 7.14 A 45° LPO below diaphragm.

- Abduct downside arm away from thorax; elevate opposite arm away from thorax.
- Align a plane of the thorax midway between the spine and the lateral margin of thorax on side of interest to CR and to midline of the grid or table/bucky.

Central Ray: CR ⊥ to IR, centered to level midway between xiphoid process and lower rib margin

SID: 72 inches (180 cm) erect, 40 inches (100 cm) recumbent

Collimation Field Size: Collimate on four sides to area of interest to include soft tissue margins

Respiration: Below diaphragm—expose upon **expiration**.

	cm	kVp	mA	Time	mAs	SID	Exposure Indicator
kVp Range:					75–85		
S							
M							
L							

Textbook, 11th ed, p. 380

Bony Thorax

7

Anterior or Posterior Oblique: Axillary Ribs
Above and Below Diaphragm

Evaluation Criteria
Anatomy Demonstrated

- **LPO/RAO:** Visualizes (elongates) left axillary ribs
- **RPO/LAO:** Visualizes (elongates) right axillary ribs
- Ribs 1–9 seen above diaphragm
- Ribs 10–12 seen below diaphragm (minimum)
- Axillary portion of ribs projected without superimposition

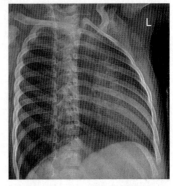

Fig. 7.15 LPO above diaphragm.

Position

- A 45° oblique should allow visualization of the axillary ribs in profile with spine shifted away from area of interest

Exposure

- Optimal image receptor exposure and contrast visualizes ribs through lungs and heart shadow for above diaphragm, and through dense abdominal organs for below diaphragm; no motion
- Sharp bony margins

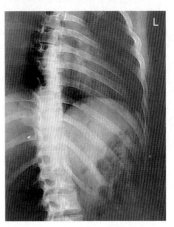

Fig. 7.16 LPO below diaphragm.

Cranium, Facial Bones, and Paranasal Sinuses

(R) Routine, (S) Special

8

Cranial Positioning Lines and Landmarks

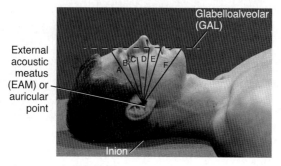

Fig. 8.1 Positioning lines.

A. Glabellomeatal line (**GML**)
B. Orbitomeatal line (**OML**)
C. Infraorbitomeatal line (**IOML**) (Reid's base line, or "base line," base of cranium)
D. Acanthiomeatal line (**AML**)
E. Lips-meatal line (**LML**) (used for modified Waters)
F. Mentomeatal line (**MML**) (used for Waters)

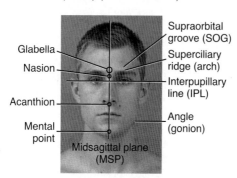

Fig. 8.2 Cranial landmarks.

- **Common positioning errors:** Rotation, tilt, excessive neck flexion and extension, and incorrect CR angle errors are the most common seen with cranial and facial bone radiography. See pp. 416 and 417 in the text to review these positioning errors and corrections.

Remove all metal, plastic, or other removable objects from the patient's head.

AP Axial: Cranium
Towne Method

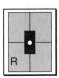

- 10 × 12 inches (24 × 30 cm), portrait
- Grid

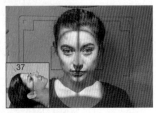

Fig. 8.3 AP axial (Towne)—CR 30° caudad to OML.

Position

- Remove all metal, plastic, or other removable objects from the patient's head.
- Patient should be seated erect or supine, MSP aligned to CR and midline of the table or IR, perpendicular to IR; no rotation or tilt.
- Depress chin to bring OML or IOML perpendicular to IR.
- Ensure that **no head rotation or tilt** exists.
- Center IR to projecting CR.

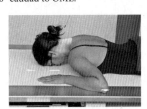

Fig. 8.4 PA axial (Haas method), OML ⊥ CR 25° cephalad, through level of EAMs.

Central Ray

- CR 30° caudal to OML; or 37° caudal to IOML
- CR directed to ≈2.5 inches (6.5 cm) above glabella (through 0.75 inch [2 cm] glabella to pass through the foramen magnum at the level of the base of the occiput)

SID: 40 inches (100 cm)

Collimation Field Size: Collimation on four sides to area of interest to include soft tissue margins

Respiration: Suspend during exposure.

Note: The PA axial—Haas method (p. 428 in text) is an alternative to AP Towne. Adjust the head to bring OML ⊥ to IR. CR is angled 25° cephalad and exits 1.5 inches (4 cm) superior to the nasion.

	cm	kVp	mA	Time	mAs	SID	Exposure Indicator
kVp Range:					75–90		
S							
M							
L							

Textbook, 11th ed, p. 423

AP Axial (Towne Method): Cranium

Evaluation Criteria

Anatomy Demonstrated

- Occipital bone, petrous pyramids, and foramen magnum are demonstrated with the dorsum sellae and posterior clinoid processes visualized in the shadow of the foramen magnum.

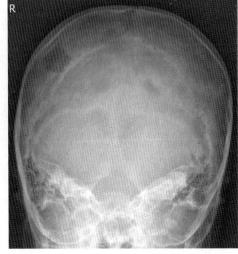

Fig. 8.5 AP axial cranium. (From Curtis: *Online course for Mosby's digital positioning consult*, Philadelphia, 2019, Elsevier.)

Position

- Petrous ridges should be symmetric, indicating **no rotation** (petrous ridge will appear narrowed in the direction of rotation).
- Dorsum sellae and posterior clinoid processes visualized in the foramen magnum indicate **correct CR angle and proper neck flexion/extension**.

Exposure

- Optimal image receptor exposure and contrast allow visualization of occipital bone and structures within foramen magnum; no motion
- Sharp bony margins

Lateral: Cranium

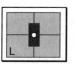

- 10 × 12 inches (24 × 30 cm), landscape
- Grid

Position
- Remove all metal, plastic, or other removable objects from patient's head.
- Patient should be seated erect or semiprone on table.
- Head should be in the true lateral position, with the

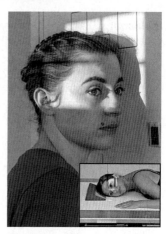

Fig. 8.6 Lateral cranium.

side of interest closest to IR, no rotation or tilt, MSP parallel to IR, and IPL perpendicular to IR.
- Adjust chin to place IOML ⊥ to front edge of IR (GAL is parallel to front edge of IR).
- Center IR to CR.

Central Ray: CR ⊥ to IR, ≈2 inches (5 cm) superior to EAM
SID: 40 inches (100 cm)
Collimation Field Size: Collimate on four sides to area of interest to include soft tissue margins
Respiration: Suspend during exposure.

	cm	kVp	mA	Time	mAs	SID	Exposure Indicator
S							
M							
L							

kVp Range: 70–85

Textbook, 11th ed, p. 424

Lateral: Cranium

Evaluation Criteria

Anatomy Demonstrated

- Entire cranium visualized and superimposed parietal bones of cranium
- Entire sella turcica and dorsum sellae

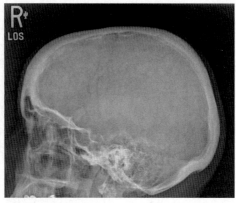

Fig. 8.7 Lateral cranium.

Position

- **No tilt**, evident by superimposition of orbital plates (roofs)
- **No rotation**, evident by superimposition of greater wings of sphenoid and mandibular rami

Exposure

- Optimal image receptor exposure and contrast allow visualization of sellar structures; no motion
- Sharp bony margins

PA and PA Axial (15°): Cranium
Caldwell Method

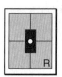

Note: Some departmental routines include a PA to better demonstrate the frontal bone in addition to the 15° PA axial (Caldwell).
- 10 × 12 inches (24 × 30 cm), portrait
- Grid

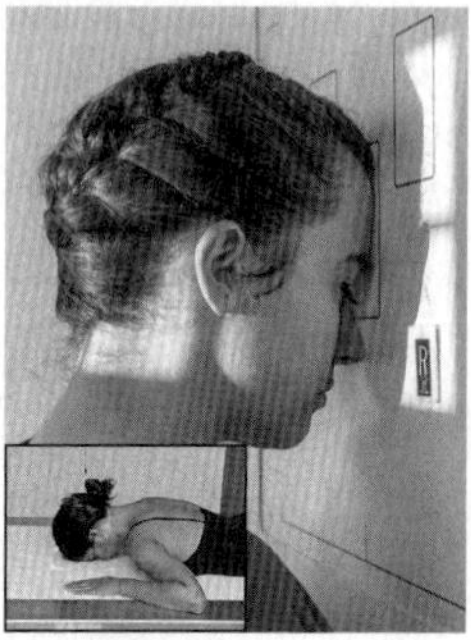

Fig. 8.8 PA—0°.

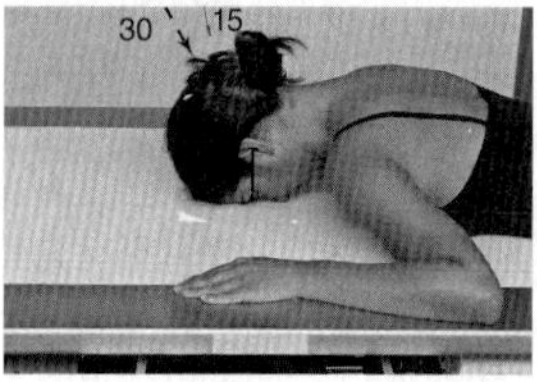

Position

- Remove all metallic or plastic objects from the patient's head and neck.
- Patient should be seated erect, or prone on the table, head aligned to CR and midline of the table or IR.
- Place patient's nose and forehead against table/imaging device surface, and adjust head to align OML perpendicular to IR.

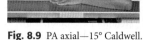

Fig. 8.9 PA axial—15° Caldwell.

- No rotation or tilt is needed; MSP should be perpendicular to IR.
- Center IR to projected CR.

Central Ray

- **PA:** CR ⊥ to IR, centered to exit at glabella
- **PA axial (Caldwell):** CR 15° caudad to OML, centered to exit at nasion (25°–30° caudad best demonstrates orbital margins)

SID: 40 inches (100 cm)

Collimation Field Size: Collimate on four sides to area of interest to include soft tissue margins

Respiration: Suspend during exposure.

	cm	kVp	mA	Time	mAs	SID	Exposure Indicator
kVp Range:					75–85		
S							
M							
L							

Textbook, 11th ed, p. 425

PA and PA Axial (15°): Cranium
Caldwell Method

Evaluation Criteria
Anatomy Demonstrated

- **PA:** Frontal bone, crista galli, internal auditory canals, frontal and anterior ethmoid sinuses, petrous ridges, greater and lesser wings of sphenoid, and dorsum sellae are demonstrated without distortion.

- **PA axial 15°:** Frontal bone, greater/lesser sphenoid wings, superior orbital fissures, frontal and anterior ethmoid sinuses, supraorbital margins, and crista galli are demonstrated.

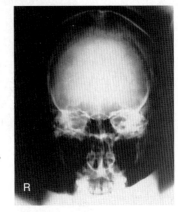

Fig. 8.10 PA—0°.

Position

- **PA:** Petrous ridges at level of superior orbital margin; no rotation; equal distance between orbits and lateral cranium

- **PA axial 15°:** Petrous ridges projected in lower one-third of orbits; no rotation; equal distance between orbits and lateral cranium

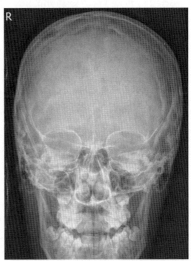

Fig. 8.11 PA axial—15° Caldwell. (From Curtis: *Online course for Mosby's digital positioning consult*, Philadelphia, 2019, Elsevier.)

Exposure

- Optimal image receptor exposure and contrast allow visualization of frontal bone and surrounding structures; no motion
- Sharp bony margins

Submentovertical (SMV): Cranium

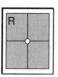

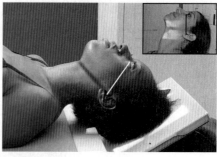

Warning: Rule out cervical spine fracture or subluxation on trauma patient before attempting this projection.

Fig. 8.12 SMV—CR ⊥ to IOML.

- 10 × 12 inches (24 × 30 cm), portrait
- Grid
- AEC optional

Position

- Remove all metal, plastic, and other removable objects from patient's head.
- Patient should be seated erect or supine with head extended over end of table, resting top of head against grid IR (may tilt table up slightly). A positioning sponge/pillow may be placed under shoulders.
- Adjust IR and hyperextend neck to place IOML parallel to IR.
- Ensure no rotation or tilt.
- Center IR to CR.

Central Ray: CR angled to be ⊥ to IOML, centered to 1.5 inches (4 cm) inferior to mandibular symphysis, or midway between the gonions (approximately 0.75 inch [2 cm] anterior to level of EAM)
Note: If patient cannot extend head this far, adjust CR as needed to remain perpendicular to IOML.
SID: 40 inches (100 cm)
Collimation Field Size: Collimate on four sides to area of interest to include soft tissue margins
Respiration: Suspend during exposure.

kVp Range:						75–85	
	cm	kVp	mA	Time	mAs	SID	Exposure Indicator
S							
M							
L							

Textbook, 11th ed, p. 427

SMV: Cranium

Evaluation Criteria

Anatomy Demonstrated

- Foramen ovale and spinosum, mandible, sphenoid and posterior ethmoid sinuses, mastoid processes, petrous ridges, hard palate, foramen magnum, and occipital bone

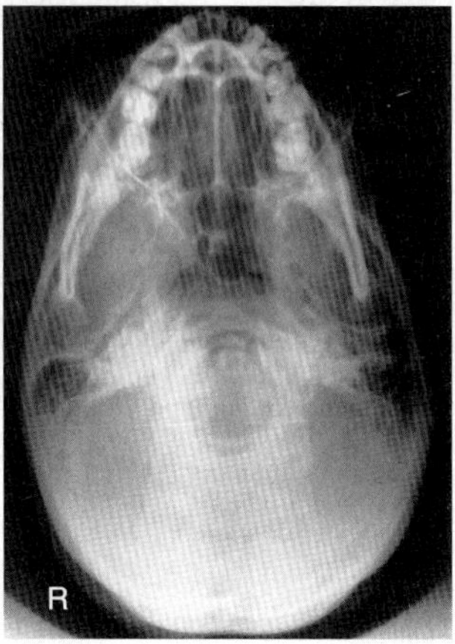

Position

- Correct extension of neck and relationship between IOML and CR as indicated by mandibular mentum anterior to the ethmoid sinuses
- **No rotation;** MSP parallel to edge of IR
- **No tilt;** equal distance between mandibular ramus and lateral cranial cortex

Fig. 8.13 SMV.

Exposure

- Optimal image receptor exposure and contrast allow visualization of outline of foramen magnum; no motion
- Sharp bony margins

Lateral: Cranium (Trauma)

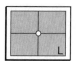

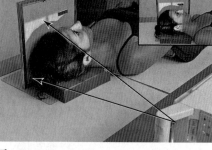

Warning: Do **NOT** elevate or move the patient's head before cervical spine injuries have been ruled out.

Fig. 8.14 Lateral, with possible spinal injury.

- 10 × 12 inches (24 × 30 cm), landscape (aligned to the anterior-to-posterior dimension of the cranium)
- Grid

Position

- Remove all metallic or plastic objects from head and neck.
- Patient should be supine; do not remove cervical collar unless instructed by physician.
- With possible spinal injury, move patient to back edge of table and place IR about 1 inch (2.5 cm) below tabletop and posterior cranium (move floating tabletop forward).
- Place head in true lateral position.
- Center IR to horizontal beam CR (to include entire cranium).
- Ensure no rotation or tilt.

Central Ray: CR horizontal, $\perp$ to IR, centered to ≈2 inches (5 cm) superior to EAM

SID: 40 inches (100 cm)

Collimation Field Size: Collimate on four sides to area of interest to include soft tissue margins

Respiration: Suspend respiration.

	cm	kVp	mA	Time	mAs	SID	Exposure Indicator
kVp Range:						70–85	
S							
M							
L							

Textbook, 11th ed, p. 601

8

Lateral: Cranium (Trauma)

Evaluation Criteria

Anatomy Demonstrated

- Entire cranium and superimposed cranial halves
- Entire sella turcica and dorsum sellae

Position

- No rotation or tilt (see p. 430 for specific criteria)

Exposure

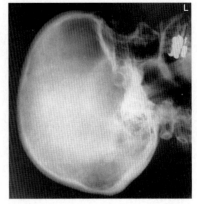

Fig. 8.15 Lateral trauma cranium.

- Optimal density (brightness) and contrast allow visualization of sellar structures; no motion
- Sharp bony margins

AP and AP Axial: Cranium (Trauma)

Warning: With possible spine or severe head injuries, perform all projections AP without moving patient's head or without removing cervical collar unless requested to do so by physician.

- 10 × 12 inches (24 × 30 cm), portrait
- Grid

Position

- Remove all metallic or plastic objects from head and neck. Do not remove cervical collar unless instructed by physician.
- Patient should be carefully moved onto x-ray table in supine position.
- All projections are performed as is without moving patient's head.

SID: 40 inches (100 cm)

Collimation Field Size: Collimate on four sides to area of interest to include soft tissue margins

Respiration: Suspend during exposure.

CR Angle and Centering

- As indicated in Figs. 8.16, 8.17, and 8.18
- IR centered to projected CR

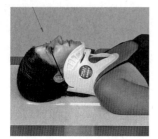

Fig. 8.16 AP, CR—parallel to OML—centered to glabella.

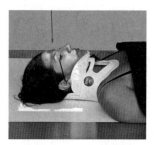

Fig. 8.17 AP reverse Caldwell. CR—15° cephalad to OML—centered to nasion.

Cranium, Facial Bones, and Paranasal Sinuses

8

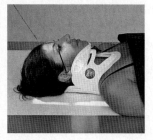

Fig. 8.18 AP axial (Towne) . CR—30° caudad to OML—CR to ≈2 .5 inches (5–6 cm) above glabella..

	cm	kVp	mA	Time	mAs	SID	Exposure Indicator
S							
M							
L							

kVp Range: 75–90

Textbook, 11th ed, pp. 602 and 603

AP and AP Axial: Cranium (Trauma)

Evaluation Criteria

Anatomy Demonstrated

- **AP 0°:** Frontal bone and crista galli demonstrated (magnified due to OID)
- **AP axial 15°:** Greater/lesser wings of sphenoid, frontal bone, and superior orbital fissures

Position

- **AP 0°:** Petrous ridges at level of superior orbital margin; **no rotation;** equal distance between orbits and lateral cranium
- **AP axial 15°:** Petrous ridges projected in lower one-third of orbits; **no rotation;** equal distance between orbits and lateral cranium

Exposure

- Optimal image receptor exposure and contrast allow visualization of frontal bone and surrounding structures; no motion
- Sharp bony margins

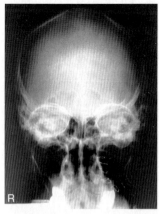

Fig. 8.19 AP to OML.

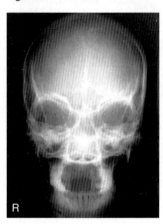

Fig. 8.20 AP axial ("reverse" Caldwell) (15° cephalad).

Lateral: Facial Bones

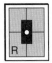

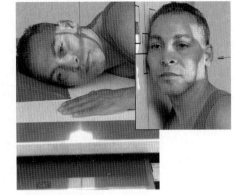

Fig. 8.21 Lateral facial bones.

- 8 × 10 inches (18 × 24 cm), portrait
- Grid

Position

- Remove all metallic or plastic objects from head and neck.
- Patient should be erect or semiprone on table.
- Rest lateral aspect of head against table or upright imaging device surface, **with side of interest closest to IR**.
- Adjust head to true lateral position (oblique body as needed for patient's comfort).
- No rotation or tilt needed; MSP should be parallel to IR, IPL perpendicular to IR.
- Adjust chin to place IOML ⊥ to front edge of IR.
- Center IR to CR.

Central Ray: CR ⊥ to IR, to zygoma (prominence of the cheek) midway between EAM and outer canthus

SID: 40 inches (100 cm)

Collimation Field Size: Collimate on four sides to area of interest to include soft tissue margins

Respiration: Suspend during exposure.

	cm	kVp	mA	Time	mAs	SID	Exposure Indicator
kVp Range:				70–85			
S							
M							
L							

Textbook, 11th ed, p. 429

Lateral: Facial Bones

Evaluation Criteria

Anatomy Demonstrated:
Superimposed facial
bones, greater wings of
sphenoid, orbital plates,
sella turcica, zygoma,
and mandible

Position
- **No tilt;** evident by
  superimposition of
  orbital plates (roofs)
- **No rotation;** evident
  by superimposition of
  greater wings of sphe-
  noid and mandibular
  rami

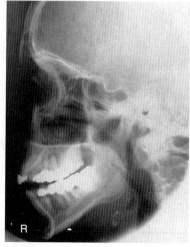

Fig. 8.22 Lateral facial bones.

Exposure
- Optimal image receptor exposure and contrast allow visualiza-
  tion of facial structures; no motion
- Sharp bony margins

Parietoacanthial: Facial Bones
Waters and Modified Waters Methods

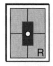

- 8 × 10 inches (18 × 24 cm), portrait, or 10 × 12 inches (24 × 30 cm), portrait
- Grid

Position
Waters
- Remove all metallic or plastic objects from head and neck.
- Patient should be seated or erect (preferred) or prone on table.
- Extend neck, resting on chin against table/upright imaging device surface; place MML ⊥ to IR, which places the OML 37° to IR.
- Center IR to CR.

Modified Waters
- OML is 55° to the plane of the IR, or line from junction of lips to EAM (LML) is ⊥ to IR.

Central Ray: CR ⊥ to IR, to exit at acanthion (both projections)
SID: 40 inches (100 cm)
Collimation Field Size: Collimate on four sides to area of interest to include soft tissue margins
Respiration: Suspend during exposure.

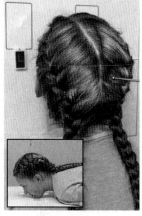

Fig. 8.23 PA Waters, OML 37°—CR and MML ⊥.

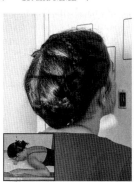

Fig. 8.24 PA modified Waters, OML 55°—CR and LML ⊥.

Cranium, Facial Bones, and Paranasal Sinuses

8

kVp Range:					70–85 kVp		
	cm	kVp	mA	Time	mAs	SID	Exposure Indicator
S							
M							
L							

Textbook, 11th ed, pp. 430 and 432

Parietoacanthial and Modified Parietoacanthial Waters and Modified Waters Methods

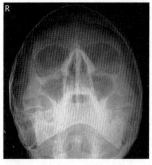

Fig. 8.25 PA Waters. (From Curtis: *Online course for Mosby's digital positioning consult*, Philadelphia, 2019, Elsevier.)

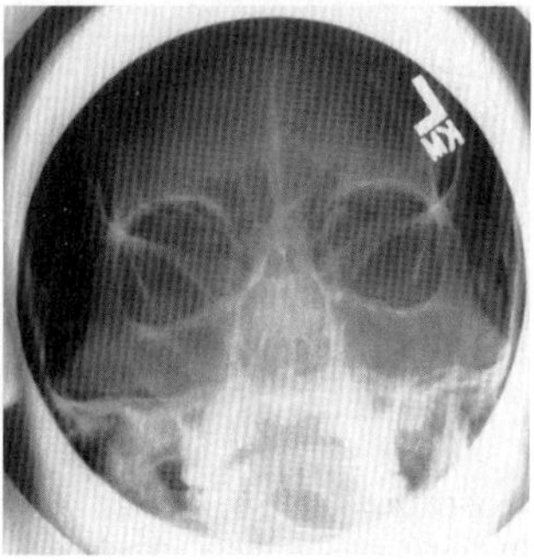

Fig. 8.26 PA modified Waters.

Evaluation Criteria

Anatomy Demonstrated

- **Waters:** IOMs, maxillae, nasal septum, zygomatic bones, zygomatic arches, and anterior nasal spine
- **Modified Waters:** Inferior orbital floors in profile (undistorted); ideal projection to demonstrate possible "blowout" fractures of orbital floor

Position

- **Waters:** Petrous ridges just inferior to floor of maxillary sinuses; **no rotation;** equal distance between orbits and lateral cranium
- **Modified Waters:** Petrous ridges projected in lower one-half of maxillary sinuses; **no rotation;** equal distance between orbits and lateral cranium

Exposure

- Optimal image receptor exposure and contrast allow visualization of maxillary region and surrounding structures; no motion
- Sharp bony margins

PA Axial (15°): Facial Bones
Caldwell Method

- 8 × 10 inches (18 × 24 cm), portrait, or 10 × 12 inches (24 × 30 cm), portrait
- Grid

Position

- Remove all metallic or plastic objects from head and neck.
- Patient should be seated erect (preferred) or prone on table, MSP aligned to CR and to midline of the table or IR.

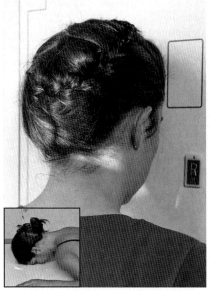

Fig. 8.27 PA axial—15° Caldwell (OML ⊥); CR to exit at nasion.

- Rest patient's nose and forehead against the imaging device, adjust head to place OML perpendicular to IR; ensure no rotation or tilt.
- Center IR to projected CR (to nasion).

Central Ray: CR 15° caudal to OML, centered to exit at nasion

Note: A 30° CR angle is required to project petrous ridges below lower orbital margins if this is an area of interest. CR will exit at level of midorbits.

SID: 40 inches (100 cm)

Collimation Field Size: Collimate on four sides to area of interest to include soft tissue margins

Respiration: Suspend during exposure.

	cm	kVp	mA	Time	mAs	SID	Exposure Indicator
S							
M							
L							

kVp Range: 70–85

Textbook, 11th ed, p. 431

8

PA Axial (15°): Facial Bones
Caldwell Method

Evaluation Criteria
Anatomy Demonstrated

- Superior orbital margins, maxillae, nasal septum, zygomatic arches, and anterior nasal spine

Position

- Petrous ridges projected in lower one-third of orbits; **no rotation;** equal distance between orbits and lateral cranial margins

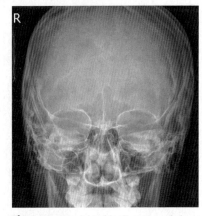

Fig. 8.28 PA axial Caldwell—15° caudad. (From Curtis: *Online course for Mosby's digital positioning consult*, Philadelphia, 2019, Elsevier.)

Exposure

- Optimal image receptor exposure and contrast. Allow visualization of maxillary region and orbital floor; no motion
- Sharp bony margins

Lateral, Acanthioparietal: Facial Bones (Trauma)
Reverse Waters and Reverse Modified Waters Methods

Warning: With possible spine or severe head injuries, perform all projections with the patient supine. Do not move the patient's head or remove the cervical collar, if present.

Lateral (Horizontal Beam)
- 8 × 10 inches (18 × 24 cm), portrait
- Grid, placed on edge against lateral cranium
- No rotation or tilt, MSP parallel to IR
- CR horizontal, to midway between outer canthus and EAM

Reverse Waters
- 8 × 10 inches (18 × 24 cm), portrait
- Grid (AEC—center chamber)
- MSP aligned to CR and midline of table or IR
- No rotation or tilt
- CR parallel to MML
- CR centered to acanthion (CR angled cephalad, as needed, unless cervical injury has been ruled out)

Reverse Modified Waters
- Same as reverse Waters except:
  - CR parallel to junction of lips-meatal line (LML)
  - CR centered to acanthion

Textbook, 11th ed, pp. 604 and 605.

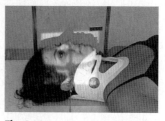

Fig. 8.29 Horizontal beam lateral—CR to midway between outer canthus and EAM.

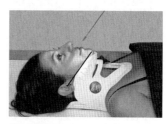

Fig. 8.30 Trauma reverse Waters—CR parallel to MML, centered to acanthion.

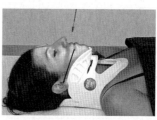

Fig. 8.31 Trauma reverse modified Waters—CR parallel to LML, centered to acanthion.

Cranium, Facial Bones, and Paranasal Sinuses

8

Lateral: Nasal Bones

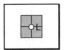

Bilateral projections generally imaged for comparison.

- 8 × 10 inches (18 × 24 cm), landscape
- Nongrid
- AEC not recommended

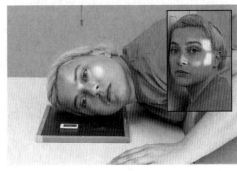

Fig. 8.32 Left lateral—nasal bones.

Position

- Remove all metallic or plastic objects from head and neck.
- Patient should be seated erect or semiprone on table.
- Rest lateral aspect of head against the table/upright imaging device surface, with side of interest closest to IR.
- Center nasal bones to center of IR.
- Adjust head into a true lateral position and oblique body as needed for patient's comfort.
- MSP should be parallel and IPL ⊥ to table/upright imaging device surface with IOML ⊥ to front edge of IR.

Central Ray: CR ⊥ to IR, centered to ≈0.5 inch (1.25 cm) inferior to nasion

SID: 40 inches (100 cm)

Collimation Field Size: Collimate on four sides to area of interest to include soft tissue margins

Respiration: Suspend during exposure.

kVp Range:				65–80			
	cm	kVp	mA	Time	mAs	SID	Exposure Indicator
S							
M							
L							

Textbook, 11th ed, p. 433

Lateral: Nasal Bones

Evaluation Criteria

Anatomy Demonstrated

- Nasal bones with soft tissue nasal structures, the frontonasal suture, and the anterior nasal spine demonstrated

Position

- **No rotation;** complete profile of nasal bones

Exposure

- Optimal image receptor exposure and contrast allow visualization of nasal bones and surrounding soft tissue structures; no motion
- Sharp bony margins with soft tissue detail

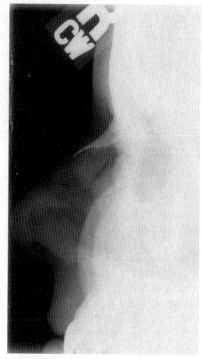

Fig. 8.33 Lateral nasal bones. (From Curtis: *Online course for Mosby's digital positioning consult*, Philadelphia, 2019, Elsevier.)

8

Superoinferior Tangential (Axial): Nasal Bones

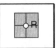

- 8 × 10 inches (18 × 24 cm), landscape
- Nongrid

Position

- Remove all metallic or plastic objects from head and neck.

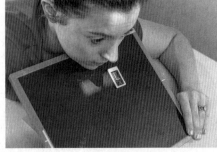

Fig. 8.34 Axial nasal bones.

- Patient should be seated erect at end of table or prone on table.
- If prone, place supports under chest and under IR.
- Rest extended chin on IR, which should be perpendicular to GAL and to CR.

Central Ray: CR directed nasion and angle as needed to ensure CR is parallel to GAL. (CR must skim glabella and anterior upper front teeth.)

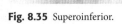

Fig. 8.35 Superoinferior.

SID: 40 inches (100 cm)

Collimation Field Size: Collimate on four sides to area of interest (≈4 inches [10 cm]) square to include soft tissue margins

Respiration: Suspend during exposure.

	cm	kVp	mA	Time	mAs	SID	Exposure Indicator
kVp Range:					65–80		
S							
M							
L							

Textbook, 11th ed, p. 434

Bilateral SMV: Zygomatic Arches

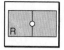

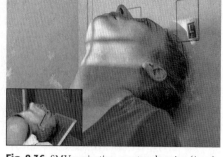

- 10 × 12 inches (24 × 30 cm), landscape
- Grid > 4 inches (10 cm)
- AEC not recommended

Fig. 8.36 SMV projection, erect and supine (*inset*)—IOML parallel to IR; CR perpendicular to IOML.

Position

- Remove all metallic or plastic objects from head and neck.
- Patient should be seated erect or supine with head extended over end of table resting top of head against grid IR (table may be tilted up slightly).
- Adjust IR and head to place IOML parallel to IR.
- Ensure no rotation or tilt.
- Center IR to CR.

Central Ray: CR angled as needed to be ⊥ to IOML, centered to midway between zygomatic arches (≈1.5 inches or 4 cm inferior to mandibular symphysis)

SID: 40 inches (100 cm)

Collimation Field Size: Collimate on four sides to area of interest to include soft tissue margins

Respiration: Suspend during exposure.

	cm	kVp	mA	Time	mAs	SID	Exposure Indicator
kVp Range:				75–85			
S							
M							
L							

Textbook, 11th ed, p. 435

Oblique Inferosuperior (Tangential): Zygomatic Arches

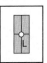

Bilateral arches generally imaged for comparison.

- 8 × 10 inches (18 × 24 cm), portrait
- Grid > 4 inches (10 cm)
- AEC not recommended

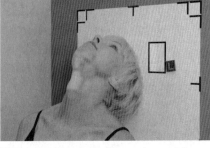

Fig. 8.37 Oblique inferosuperior (tangential), upright imaging device (15° tilt, 15° rotation, CR perpendicular to IOML).

Position

- Remove all metallic or plastic objects from head and neck.
- Patient should be erect (preferred) or supine; position as for an SMV cranium with the IOML parallel to the IR.
- **Rotate** the head ≈15° **toward** side being examined.
- **Tilt** the chin MSP ≈15° **toward** side of interest (more tilt may be needed to free the zygomatic arch from superimposition by mandible or parietal bone).
- Center IR to CR.

Central Ray: CR angled if needed to be ⊥ to IOML, centered to zygomatic arch. (CR skims mandibular ramus, passes through arch, and parietal eminence on the downside.)

SID: 40 inches (100 cm)

Collimation Field Size: Collimate on four sides to area of interest to include soft tissue margins

Respiration: Suspend during exposure.

	cm	kVp	mA	Time	mAs	SID	Exposure Indicator
S							
M							
L							

kVp Range: 70–85

Textbook, 11th ed, p. 436

SMV and Oblique Inferosuperior (Tangential): Zygomatic Arches

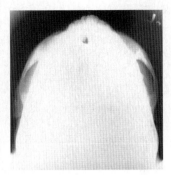

Fig. 8.38 SMV.

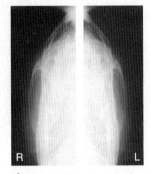

Fig. 8.39 Oblique tangential.

Evaluation Criteria

Anatomy Demonstrated
- **SMV:** Bilateral zygomatic arches
- **Tangential:** Unilateral zygomatic arch

Position
- **SMV:** Unobstructed view of bilateral arches; no rotation; symmetry of arches
- **Oblique inferosuperior (tangential):** Unilateral view of unobstructed arch; no superimposition of arch with parietal bone or mandible

Exposure
- Optimal image receptor exposure and contrast allow visualization of the zygomatic arches; no motion
- Sharp bony margins with soft tissue detail

AP Axial: Zygomatic Arches
Modified Towne Method

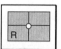

- 8 × 10 inches (18 × 24 cm), landscape
- Grid
- AEC not recommended

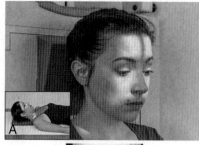

Position

- Remove all metallic or plastic objects from head and neck.
- Patient should be seated erect or

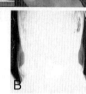

Fig. 8.40 AP axial—zygomatic arches—CR 30° to OML(37° to IOML), erect and supine (*inset*).

supine on table, MSP aligned to midline of table/upright imaging device surface to prevent head rotation or tilt.
- Flex neck to bring chin to place the OML or the IOML perpendicular to IR.
- Center IR to projected CR.

Central Ray

- CR 30° caudad to OML; or 37° to IOML
- CR 1 inch (2.5 cm) superior to nasion (to pass through midarches) at level of the gonion

SID: 40 inches (100 cm)

Collimation Field Size: Collimate on four sides to area of interest to include soft tissue margins

Respiration: Suspend during exposure.

kVp Range:						70–85	
	cm	kVp	mA	Time	mAs	SID	Exposure Indicator
S							
M							
L							

Textbook, 11th ed, p. 437

Parieto-Oribital Oblique: Optic Foramina
Rhese Method

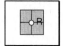

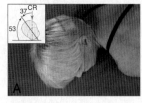
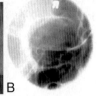

- 8 × 10 inches (18 × 24 cm), landscape
- Grid
- Bilateral orbit study imaged for comparison
- AEC not recommended

Fig. 8.41 (A) Rhese oblique (right side). (B) Rhese oblique. —AML and CR ⊥ —53° rotation of head from lateral.

Position

- Remove all metallic or plastic objects from the head and neck.
- Patient should be seated erect or prone on table.
- As a starting reference, position patient's head in a prone position with MSP perpendicular to IR. Adjust flexion and extension so that AML is perpendicular to the IR. Adjust the patient's head so that the chin, cheek, and nose touch the table/upright imaging device surface (this position is historically known as the "3 point landing").
- Rotate the head 37° toward the affected side. The angle formed between MSP and plane of IR measures 53°. (An angle indicator should be used to obtain an accurate angle of 37° from CR to MSP.)
- Center IR to CR (to downside orbit).

Central Ray: CR ⊥ to IR, to midportion of downside orbit
SID: 40 inches (100 cm)
Collimation Field Size: Closely collimate on four sides to area of interest (to 3–4 inches [8–10 cm]) to include soft tissue margins.
Respiration: Suspend during exposure.

	cm	kVp	mA	Time	mAs	SID	Exposure Indicator
S							
M							
L							

kVp Range: 70–85

Textbook, 11th ed, p. 438

8

PA and PA Axial: Mandible

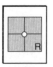

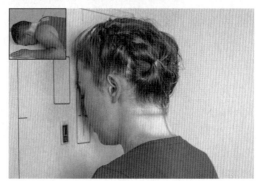

Fig. 8.42 PA mandible—CR and OML ⊥ to IR.

- 8 × 10 inches (18 × 24 cm), or 10 × 12 inches (24 × 30 cm), portrait
- Grid (often performed nongrid)
- AEC not recommended

Position

- Remove all metallic or plastic objects from head and neck
- Patient should be seated erect or prone on table, head aligned to midline of the table or IR.
- Place head in a true lateral position, with side of interest against IR.
- With forehead and nose resting on tabletop, adjust head to place OML ⊥ to IR.
- No rotation or tilt needed; MSP ⊥ to IR.
- Center IR to CR (level of junction of lips).

Central Ray: CR ⊥ to IR, to exit mandibular region of interest

PA Axial (Optional): A CR angle of 20°–25° cephalad centered to exit at the acanthion best demonstrates proximal rami and condyles.

SID: 40 inches (100 cm)

Collimation Field Size: Collimate on four sides to area of interest to include soft tissue margins

Respiration: Suspend during exposure.

	cm	kVp	mA	Time	mAs	SID	Exposure Indicator
kVp Range:					75–90		
S							
M							
L							

Textbook, 11th ed, p. 441

8

Axiolateral and Axiolateral Oblique: Mandible

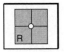

Fig. 8.43 Semisupine.

R and L sides are generally imaged for comparison unless contraindicated.

- 8 × 10 inches (18 × 24 cm) or 10 × 12 inches (24 × 30 cm), landscape
- Grid >4 inches (10 cm)
- AEC not recommended

Position

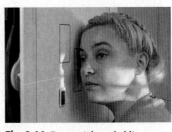

Fig. 8.44 Erect axiolateral oblique. — CR 25° cephalad (maximum) —10°–15° head rotation for general survey (as shown above) —0° head rotation for ramus —30° head rotation for body —45° head rotation for mentum.

- Remove all metallic or plastic objects from head and neck.
- Patient should be seated erect, semiprone, or semisupine, with support under shoulder and hip.
- Extend chin, with side of interest against IR.
- Adjust head so IPL is perpendicular to IR, no tilt.
- Rotate head toward IR as determined by area of interest:
  - Head in true lateral demonstrates ramus (axiolateral).
  - 10°–15° rotation best provides a general survey of the mandible.
  - 30° rotation toward IR best demonstrates body.
  - 45° rotation best demonstrates mentum.

Central Ray: Three methods are suggested for demonstrating the specific region of the mandible of interest (side closest to IR) without superimposing the opposite side:

1. Use CR 25° cephalad to IPL, centered to downside mid-mandible (≈2 inches or 5 cm below upside angle).
2. Employ a combination of tilt of head and CR angle not to exceed 25° cephalad (e.g., angle the tube 10° cephalad and add 15° of head tilt toward the IR).
3. Use 25° of head tilt toward IR, and use perpendicular CR.

SID: 40 inches (100 cm)

Collimation Field Size: Collimate on four sides to area of interest to include soft tissue margins

Respiration: Suspend during exposure.

kVp Range:				70–85		
	cm	kVp	mA	Time	mAs	SID	Exposure Indicator
S							
M							
L							

Cranium, Facial Bones, and Paranasal Sinuses

8

Axiolateral Oblique: Mandible (Trauma)

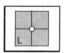

Use this method for trauma patients unable to cooperate.

- 8 × 10 inches (18 × 24 cm), or 10 × 12 inches (24 × 30 cm), landscape
- Grid > 4 inches (10 cm)

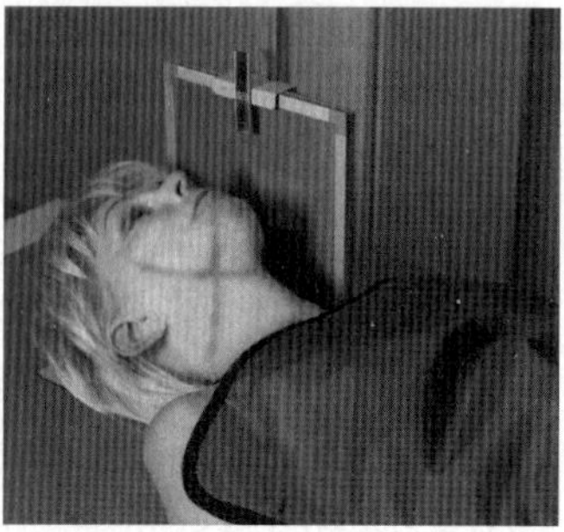

Position

- Remove all metallic or plastic objects from head and neck.

Fig. 8.45 Horizontal beam axiolateral—CR 25° cephalad from lateral, 5°–10° down.

- Patient should be supine, no rotation of head, MSP ⊥ to tabletop.
- IR should be on edge of table next to face, parallel to MSP with lower edge of IR ≈1 inch (2.5 cm) below lower border of mandible.
- Depress shoulders and elevate or extend chin, if possible.

Note: The patient's head may be rotated toward the IR slightly (10°–15°) to improve visualization of the body or the mentum of the mandible if this is an area of interest.

Central Ray

- CR horizontal beam, 25° cephalad (from lateral or IPL); angled down (posteriorly) 5°–10° to clear shoulder
- CR centered to ≈2 inches (5 cm) distal to angle of mandible on side away from IR

SID: 40 inches (100 cm)

Collimation Field Size: Collimate on four sides to area of interest to include soft tissue margins

Respiration: Suspend during exposure.

	cm	kVp	mA	Time	mAs	SID	Exposure Indicator
kVp Range:				70–85			
S							
M							
L							

Textbook, 11th ed, p. 439

PA and Axiolateral Oblique: Mandible

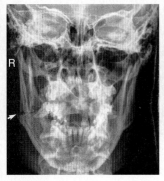

Fig. 8.46 PA mandible.

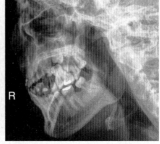

Fig. 8.47 Axiolateral oblique mandible.

Evaluation Criteria

Anatomy Demonstrated
- **PA:** Mandibular rami and lateral portion of body
- **Axiolateral and Axiolateral Oblique:** Mandibular rami, condylar and coronoid processes, and body of near side

Position
- Patient erect or supine; **PA: No rotation** evident by symmetry of rami
- **Axiolateral and Axiolateral Oblique:** Unobstructed view of mandibular rami, body, and mentum; no foreshortening of area of interest

Exposure
- Optimal image receptor exposure and contrast allow visualization of mandibular area of interest; no motion
- Sharp bony margins

8

AP Axial: Mandible or Temporomandibular Joints and Condyloid Processes

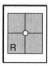

- 8 × 10 inches (18 × 24 cm), portrait
- Grid

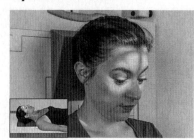

Fig. 8.48 AP axial, CR 35° to OML.

Position

- Remove all metallic or plastic objects from head and neck.
- Patient should be seated erect or supine on table, MSP centered to midline of table; ensure no rotation or tilt.
- Rest patient's posterior cranium against table/upright imaging device surface.
- Tuck chin, bringing OML perpendicular to table/imaging device surface, if possible (or place IOML perpendicular and add 7° to caudad CR angle).
- Center IR to projected CR.

Central Ray

- CR 35° caudad to OML (42° to IOML)
- Direct CR 3 inches (7.5 cm) superior to the nasion. Center IR to projected CR.

Note: CR should be centered ≈1 inch (2.5 cm) above glabella to pass through TMJs if TMJs are of primary interest.

SID: 40 inches (100 cm)

Collimation Field Size: Collimate on four sides to area of interest to include soft tissue margins

Respiration: Suspend during exposure.

kVp Range:					75–85	
	cm	kVp	mA	Time	mAs	SID	Exposure Indicator
S							
M							
L							

Textbook, 11th ed, p. 446

8

Axiolateral Oblique: Temporomandibular Joints
Modified Law Method

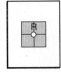

Warning: Opening the mouth should not be attempted in patients with a possible fracture.

Bilateral sides are imaged for comparison in both open- and closed-mouth positions.

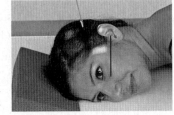

Fig. 8.49 Closed mouth.

- 8 × 10 inches (18 × 24 cm), portrait
- Grid
- AEC not recommended

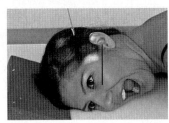

Fig. 8.50 Open mouth. —15° oblique (from lateral) and 15° CR (caudad)

Position

- Patient should be seated erect (preferred) or semi-prone on table, affected side down.
- Adjust chin to place IOML perpendicular to front edge of IR.
- From lateral position, rotate cranium (MSP) 15° toward IR, no tilt, IPL perpendicular to IR.
- Second exposure should be taken in same position except with mouth fully open.

Central Ray: CR 15° caudad, centered to enter 1.5 inches (4 cm) superior to upside EAM

SID: 40 inches (100 cm)

Collimation Field Size: Collimate on four sides to area of interest to include soft tissue margins

Respiration: Suspend during exposure.

	cm	kVp	mA	Time	mAs	SID	Exposure Indicator
kVp Range:			75–85				
S							
M							
L							

Axiolateral: Temporomandibular Joints
Schuller Method

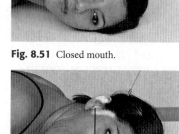

Fig. 8.51 Closed mouth.

Fig. 8.52 Open mouth. —25° caudad, 0° rotation

Warning: Opening the mouth should not be attempted in patients with possible a fracture.

Bilateral sides imaged for comparison in both open- and closed-mouth positions.

- 8 × 10 inches (18 × 24 cm), portrait
- Grid

Position

- Patient should be seated erect or semiprone, affected side down.
- Adjust head into **true lateral position**, and move patient's body in an oblique direction, as needed for patient's comfort.
- Align **IPL perpendicular** to IR.
- Align **MSP parallel** with table/imaging device surface.
- Position **IOML perpendicular** to front edge of IR.
- Second exposure should be taken in same position except with mouth fully open.

Central Ray: CR 25°–30° caudad, centered to enter 2 inches (5 cm) superior and 0.5 inch (1–2 cm) anterior to upside EAM

SID: 40 inches (100 cm)

Collimation Field Size: Collimate on four sides to area of interest to include soft tissue margins

Respiration: Suspend during exposure.

	cm	kVp	mA	Time	mAs	SID	Exposure Indicator
S							
M							
L							

kVp Range: 75–85

Cranium, Facial Bones, and Paranasal Sinuses

8

Axiolateral Oblique (Modified Law Method) and Axiolateral (Schuller Method): Temporomandibular Joints

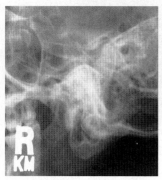

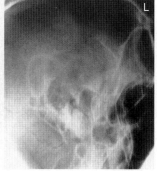

Fig. 8.53 Axiolateral oblique— closed mouth, downside TMJ shown in fossa (modified Law).

Fig. 8.54 Axiolateral projection— open mouth; TMJ shown with condyle moved to anterior margin of fossa (Schuller).

Note: Positioning routine would require both open and closed mouth of modified Law method, or both open and closed of Schuller method.

Evaluation Criteria

Anatomy Demonstrated
- Modified law: Bilateral, functional study of TMJ and fossa
- Schuller: Bilateral, functional study of TMJ and fossa

Position
- **Modified law:** Unobstructed view of TMJ in both open- and closed-mouth positions (only closed mouth is shown)
- **Schuller:** Unobstructed view of TMJ in both open- and closed-mouth positions; greater elongation of the condyles (only open mouth is shown)

Exposure
- Optimal image receptor exposure and contrast allow visualization of the TMJ and mandibular fossa; no motion
- Sharp bony margins

Lateral: Paranasal Sinuses

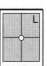

Requires an **erect position with horizontal CR** to demonstrate air-fluid levels.

Fig. 8.55 Erect lateral.

- 8 × 10 inches (18 × 24 cm), portrait
- Grid
- AEC not recommended

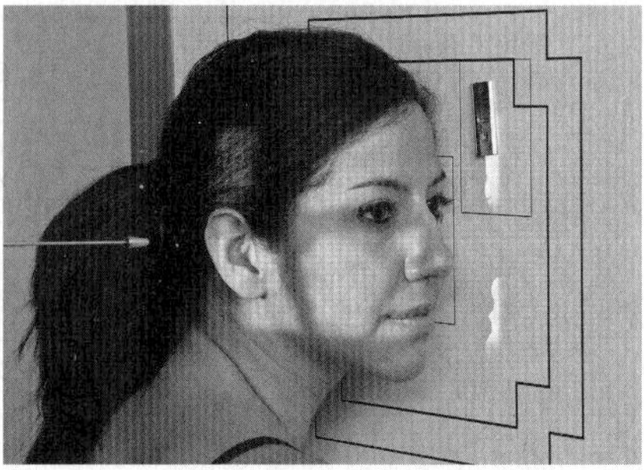

Position

- Remove all metal, plastic, and other removable objects from head.
- Patient should be erect, seated facing IR; turn head into true lateral position, moving body in an oblique direction as needed for patient's comfort, with side of interest closest to IR.
- Adjust chin to align IOML perpendicular to front edge of IR.
- No rotation needed; MSP should be parallel and IPL ⊥ to IR.
- Center IR to CR.

Central Ray: CR horizontal to midway between outer canthus and EAM

SID: 40 inches (100 cm)

Collimation Field Size: Collimate on four sides to area of interest to include soft tissue margins

Respiration: Suspend during exposure.

	cm	kVp	mA	Time	mAs	SID	Exposure Indicator
S							
M							
L							

kVp Range: 75–85

Textbook, 11th ed, p. 449

PA: Paranasal Sinuses
Modified PA–Caldwell Method

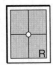

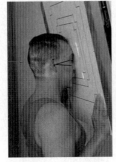

Fig. 8.56 PA Caldwell (if IR holder can be tilted).

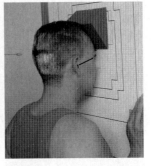

Fig. 8.57 Modified PA Caldwell (if IR holder cannot be tilted).

Requires an **erect position with horizontal CR** to demonstrate air-fluid levels.

- 8 × 10 inches (18 × 24 cm), portrait
- Grid
- AEC not recommended

Position
PA Caldwell

- Remove all metallic or plastic objects from head and neck.
- Patient should be seated erect; place patient's nose and forehead against upright imaging device or table with neck extended to elevate **OML 15° from horizontal**.
- IR should be centered to CR (nasion), no rotation.

Modified PA Caldwell

- Tilt head back to bring OML 15° from horizontal.

Central Ray: CR horizontal (parallel to floor) and exits at nasion
SID: 40 inches (100 cm)
Collimation Field Size: Collimate on four sides to area of interest to include soft tissue margins
Respiration: Suspend during exposure.

	cm	kVp	mA	Time	mAs	SID	Exposure Indicator
kVp Range:					75–85		
S							
M							
L							

Textbook, 11th ed, p. 450

Lateral and PA (Modified Caldwell Method): Sinuses

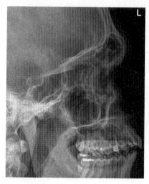

Fig. 8.58 Lateral sinuses. (From Curtis: *Online course for Mosby's digital positioning consult*, Philadelphia, 2019, Elsevier.)

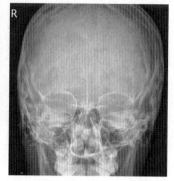

Fig. 8.59 PA axial (Caldwell method)—sinuses. (From Curtis: *Online course for Mosby's digital positioning consult*, Philadelphia, 2019, Elsevier.)

Evaluation Criteria

Anatomy Demonstrated
- **Lateral:** All paranasal sinuses demonstrated
- **PA Caldwell:** Frontal and anterior ethmoid sinuses

Position
- **Lateral: No rotation or tilt;** superimposition of greater wings/sphenoid, orbital roofs, and sella turcica
- **PA Caldwell:** Petrous ridges in lower one-third of orbits; **no rotation;** equal distance between orbits and lateral cranium

Exposure
- Optimal image receptor exposure and contrast allow visualization of the paranasal sinuses; no motion
- Sharp bony margins with soft tissue detail

Parietoacanthial: Paranasal Sinuses
Waters Method

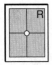

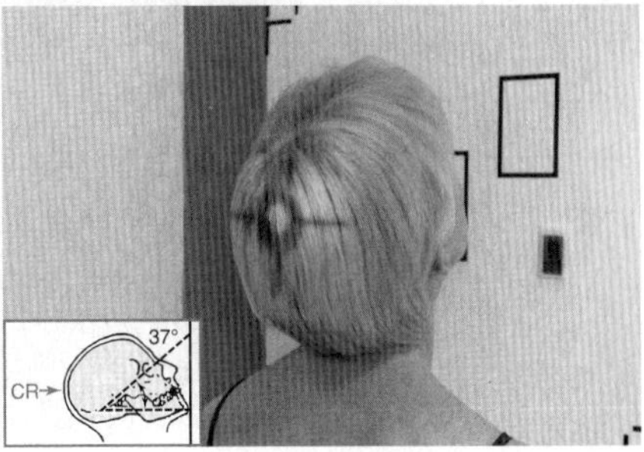

Requires an **erect position with horizontal CR** to demonstrate air-fluid levels.

- 8 × 10 inches (18 × 24 cm), or 10 × 12 inches (24 × 30 cm), portrait
- Grid
- AEC not recommended

Fig. 8.60 PA erect Waters, MML ⊥, and CR horizontal.

Position
- Remove all metallic or plastic objects from head and neck.
- Patient should be seated erect, chin and nose against table/upright imaging device surface.
- Adjust MML perpendicular to IR (OML is 37° to IR).
- No rotation needed; MSP perpendicular to IR
- Center IR to CR.

Optional Open-Mouth Position
- Patient opens mouth wide to allow better visualization of sphenoid sinuses through the open mouth.

Central Ray: CR horizontal and ⊥ to IR, to exit at acanthion
SID: 40 inches (100 cm)
Collimation Field Size: Collimate on four sides to area of interest to include soft tissue margins
Respiration: Suspend during exposure.

	cm	kVp	mA	Time	mAs	SID	Exposure Indicator
kVp Range:				75–85			
S							
M							
L							

Textbook, 11th ed, p. 451

8

SMV: Paranasal Sinuses

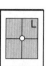

Requires an **erect position with horizontal CR** to demonstrate air-fluid levels.

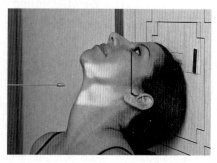

Fig. 8.61 SMV sinuses—CR ⊥ to IOML and IR.

- 8 × 10 inches (18 × 24 cm), or 10 × 12 inches (24 × 30 cm), portrait
- Grid
- AEC not recommended

Position

- Remove all metallic or plastic objects from head and neck.
- Patient should be seated erect and leaning back in chair.
- Raise chin, hyperextend neck if possible until IOML is parallel to table/upright imaging device surface.
- Head rests on vertex of cranium.
- Align MSP perpendicular to midline of the grid; ensure no rotation or tilt.
- Center IR to CR.

Central Ray: CR horizontal and ⊥ to IOML, centered to midpoint between angles of mandible at level 1.5–2 inches (4–5 cm) inferior to mandibular symphysis

SID: 40 inches (100 cm)

Collimation Field Size: Collimate on four sides to area of interest to include soft tissue margins

Respiration: Suspend during exposure.

	cm	kVp	mA	Time	mAs	SID	Exposure Indicator
S							
M							
L							

kVp Range: 75–85

Textbook, 11th ed, p. 452

Parietoacanthial (Waters Method) and SMV: Sinuses

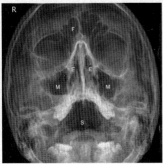

Fig. 8.62 PA Open-mouth (Waters) sinuses. (Modified from Curtis: *Online course for Mosby's digital positioning consult*, Philadelphia, 2019, Elsevier.)

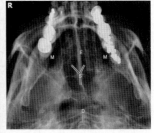

Fig. 8.63 SMV sinuses. (Modified from Curtis: *Online course for Mosby's digital positioning consult*, Philadelphia, 2019, Elsevier.)

Evaluation Criteria
Anatomy Demonstrated: Waters: Unobstructed view of maxillary sinuses

Open-mouth Waters: Sphenoid sinus projected through oral cavity

SMV: Unobstructed view of sphenoid, maxillary, and ethmoid sinuses

Position
- **Waters:** Petrous ridges just inferior to floor of maxillary sinuses; **no rotation;** equal distance between orbits and lateral cranium
- **SMV:** Mandibular condyles projected anterior to petrous bone; **no rotation or tilt;** symmetry of petrous pyramids and equal distance between mandibular border and lateral cranium

Exposure
- Optimal image receptor exposure and contrast allow visualization of the paranasal sinuses; no motion
- Sharp bony margins with soft tissue detail

Chapter 9

Abdomen and Common Contrast Media Procedures

(R) Routine, (S) Special

Abdomen and Common Contrast Media Procedures

9

Radiation Protection Principles and Practices

Abdomen and Common Contrast Media Procedures

Exposure Patterns

Fig. 9.1 reminds the technologist to not stand close to the radiographic table or either side of the fluoroscopist. It is recommended to increase distance from the higher scatter fields when possible.

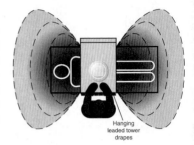

Hanging
leaded tower
drapes

Fig. 9.1 Fluoroscopy exposure patterns

Technologist Protection Devices and Dosimetry

During fluoroscopy, the technologist must wear a 0.5 mm lead equivalent (Pb/Eq) apron. Optional protective devices include Pb/Eq protective eyewear and thyroid shield. During fluoroscopy, the dosimeter should be placed at the level of the collar, outside of the lead apron (Fig. 9.2)

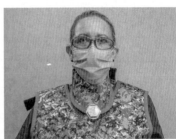

Fig. 9.2 Lead apron with thyroid shield, lead glasses and personnel dosimeter

Pregnancy and Shielding

- Generally, no radiographic procedures exposing the pelvic region should be performed during pregnancy without special instruction from a radiologist/physician. Follow department policy and protocol regarding imaging pregnant patients.
- Follow local regulations, department policy and protocol in the use of shielding.

9

Topographic Positioning Landmarks

Abdominal borders and organs within the abdomen are not visible from the exterior. We must rely on palpation of certain bony landmarks to identify the location of specific organs. There are seven landmarks of the abdomen. They include the xiphoid process (level of T9–T10), inferior costal (rib) margin (level of L2–L3), iliac crest (level of L4–L5 vertebral interspace), anterior superior iliac spine (ASIS), greater trochanter, symphysis pubis. and ischial tuberosity.

Note: Palpation must be performed gently because the patient may have painful or sensitive areas within the abdomen and pelvis. Also, ensure the patient is informed of the purpose of palpation before beginning.

Barium Distribution and Body Positions

The air-barium distribution within the stomach and large intestine changes with various body positions. By knowing these distribution patterns, one can determine the body position from which an image was taken. Air always rises to the highest levels, and the heavy barium settles to the lowest levels (air is black, and barium is white).

Stomach

The fundus is located more posteriorly; therefore, in the supine position, the fundus would be the lowest portion of the stomach and would be filled with barium.

In both prone and erect positions, the fundus would be filled with air, as seen on the drawings that follow, with a straight air-barium line demonstrated in the erect position.

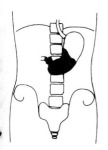 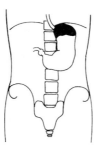 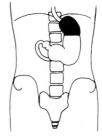

Fig. 9.3 Supine (barium in fundus).

Fig. 9.4 Prone (barium in body and pylorus).

Fig. 9.5 Erect (straight-line barium-air level). Barium = white, air = black.

Large Intestine

The ascending and descending portions are located more posteriorly, and thus more of these parts would be filled with barium (white) in the **supine position** and with air (black) in the **prone position**.

Note: This much separation of barium and air occurs generally only with double-contrast barium-air studies.

Air-fluid levels are demonstrated with the patient in the **erect position**, in which the air would rise to the highest position in each of the various sections of the large intestine, as shown in the accompanying figures.

Right and left decubitus projections (not shown on these drawings) also would demonstrate air-fluid levels, with air again rising to the highest portions.

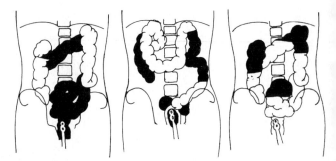

Fig. 9.6 Supine.   **Fig. 9.7** Prone.   **Fig. 9.8** Erect.

Acute Abdomen Series

Three-view abdomen:
- AP supine (KUB)
- AP erect
- PA chest

Two-view abdomen:
- AP supine (KUB)
- Left lateral decubitus

AP Supine (KUB): Abdomen (Adult)

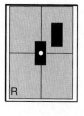

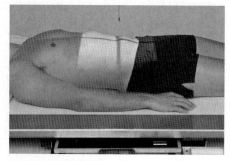

- 14 × 17 inches
  (35 × 43 cm),
  portrait
- Grid

Fig. 9.9 KUB abdomen.

Position

- Patient should be supine, legs extended, arms at sides.
- MSP should be aligned and centered to midline of table or IR.
- Ensure no rotation (ASISs equal distance from tabletop).
- Center of IR should be positioned to level of iliac crests, with bottom margin at symphysis pubis. (A hypersthenic patient may require that the IR be placed in landscape position with a second IR centered higher.)

Central Ray: CR ⊥ to center of IR (level of iliac crests)
SID: 40 inches (100 cm)
Collimation Field Size: Collimate on four sides to area of interest to include soft tissue margins
Respiration: Exposure at end of expiration

kVp Range:					70–85		
	cm	kVp	mA	Time	mAs	SID	Exposure Indicator
S							
M							
L							

Textbook, 11th ed, p. 114

AP Erect: Abdomen

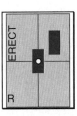

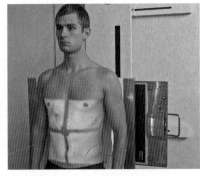

Fig. 9.10 Erect AP (include diaphragm).

- 14 × 17 inches (35 × 43 cm), portrait
- Grid
- Erect marker
- **Perform erect abdominal image first** if the patient comes to the department ambulatory or in a wheelchair in an erect position.
- Patient should be upright a minimum of **5 minutes; 10 to 20 minutes** is desirable before exposure for visualizing small amounts of intraperitoneal air.
- **Marker:** Include erect and side markers on IR.

Position

- Patient should be erect, back against table or upright IR device, arms at sides.
- MSP should be aligned and centered to centerline.
- Ensure no rotation.
- Center of IR should be ≈2 inches (5 cm) above iliac crest to include diaphragm.

Central Ray: CR horizontal, to center of IR (2 inches [5 cm] above iliac crest)

SID: 40 inches (100 cm)

Collimation Field Size: Collimate on four sides to area of interest to include soft tissue margins

Respiration: Exposure at end of expiration

	cm	kVp	mA	Time	mAs	SID	Exposure Indicator
kVp Range:				70–85			
S							
M							
L							

Textbook, 11th ed, p. 118

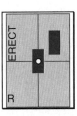 *Abdomen and Common Contrast Media Procedures*

9

AP Supine and AP Erect: Abdomen

Evaluation Criteria
Anatomy Demonstrated
- **AP supine:** Outline of liver, spleen, kidneys, psoas muscles, and air-filled stomach and bowel segments and the symphysis pubis to ensure the urinary bladder region is visualized
- **AP erect:** Air-filled stomach and loops of bowel and air-fluid levels where present
- Bilateral hemidiaphragm and as much of lower abdomen as possible

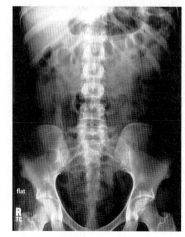

Fig. 9.11 AP KUB.

Position
- **AP supine and erect:** No rotation; symmetry of iliac wings and outer, lower rib margins

Exposure
- Optimal image receptor exposure and contrast allow visualization of psoas muscles and lumbar transverse processes; no motion.
- Air-fluid levels seen, if present

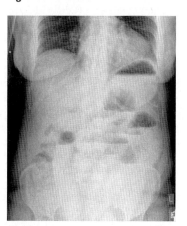

Fig. 9.12 AP erect.

- Liver margins and kidneys visible on patients of average size

Lateral Decubitus (AP): Abdomen

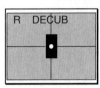

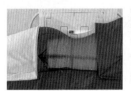

Fig. 9.13 Left lateral decubitus (AP).

- 14 × 17 inches (35 × 43 cm), landscape
- Grid
- Markers: Decubitus marker and arrow marker to indicate "up" side. Patient should be on side **a minimum of 5 minutes** before exposure; a period of **10–20 minutes is preferred**.
- Left lateral decubitus position allows best visualization of free intraperitoneal air in the area of the liver in the right upper abdomen away from the gastric bubble.

Position

- Patient should be lateral recumbent on radiolucent pad, firmly against table or vertical grid device (with wheels on cart locked so as not to move away from table).
- Patient should be on a firm surface, such as a cardiac or back board, positioned under the sheet to prevent sagging and anatomy cutoff.
- Knees should be partially flexed, arms up near head.
- Adjust patient and stretcher so that center of IR and CR is approximately 2 inches (5 cm) above level of iliac crest (to include diaphragm).
- Adjust height of IR to ensure that upside of abdomen is included for possible free air.

Central Ray: CR horizontal, to center of IR, approximately 2 inches (5 cm) above level of iliac crest; horizontal beam to demonstrate air-fluid levels and possible free intraperitoneal air
SID: 40 inches (100 cm)
Collimation Field Size: Collimate on four sides to area of interest to include soft tissue margins
Respiration: Exposure at end of expiration

	cm	kVp	mA	Time	mAs	SID	Exposure Indicator
kVp Range:				70–85			
S							
M							
L							

Dorsal Decubitus (Lateral): Abdomen

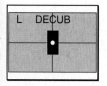

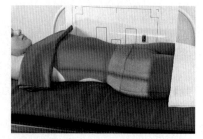

- 14 × 17 inches (35 × 43 cm), landscape
- Grid
- To include decubitus and side markers

Fig. 9.14 Dorsal decubitus (L lateral).

Position

- Patient should be supine (on decubitus board or support to elevate posterior abdomen), side against table, arms above head.
- Secure stretcher (lock wheels).
- Center IR and table (and CR) at level of iliac crest (2 inches [5 cm] above iliac crest to include diaphragm).
- Adjust height of IR to align midcoronal plane to centerline of IR.

Central Ray: CR horizontal, to center of IR at iliac crest and 2 inches (5 cm) above iliac crest to include diaphragm
SID: 40 inches (100 cm)
Collimation Field Size: Collimate on four sides to area of interest to include soft tissue margins
Respiration: Exposure at end of expiration

	cm	kVp	mA	Time	mAs	SID	Exposure Indicator
kVp Range:				70–85			
S							
M							
L							

Textbook, 11th ed, p. 119

Lateral and Dorsal Decubitus: Abdomen

Evaluation Criteria

Anatomy Demonstrated

- **Lateral decubitus:** Abdomen visualized to include air-filled stomach and bowel and upside diaphragm
- **Dorsal decubitus:** Abdomen visualized to include hemidiaphragms

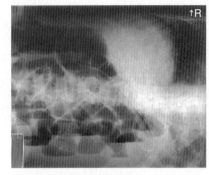

Fig. 9.15 Left lateral decubitus.

Position

- **Lateral decubitus: No rotation;** symmetry of iliac wings and spine straight
- **Dorsal decubitus: No rotation;** symmetry of iliac wings and diaphragm. Intervertebral joint spaces and vertebral bodies should be visible.

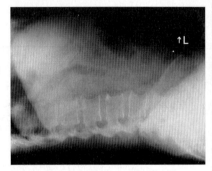

Fig. 9.16 Dorsal decubitus.

Exposure

- Optimal image receptor exposure and contrast to allow visualization of soft tissue structures and lumbar spine; no motion
- Soft tissue structures and any intraperitoneal air demonstrated on patients of average size

AP Supine (KUB): Abdomen (Pediatric)

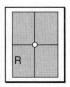

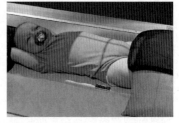

Fig. 9.17 Child AP abdomen (KUB).

- IR size determined by size of patient, portrait
- Grid > 4 inches (10 cm)
- Shortest exposure time possible

Position (Infant)
- Patient should be supine; apply immobilization as necessary.
- Center IR to CR.

Parental Assistance for Infant: Use only if necessary. Supply a lead apron and gloves, and have the parent hold the patient's arms above the head with one hand and legs with the other hand, preventing rotation.

Central Ray
- *Newborn–1 year old:* CR to 1 inch (2.5 cm) above umbilicus
- *Older child:* CR to level of iliac crest

Minimum SID: 40 inches (100 cm)

Collimation Field Size: Collimate on four sides to area of interest to include soft tissue margins

Respiration: Expose on expiration or when abdomen has least movement. If crying, time exposures at full expiration.

	cm	kVp	mA	Time	mAs	SID	Exposure Indicator
S							
M							
L							

kVp Range: 60–75

Textbook, 11th ed, p. 652

AP Erect: Abdomen (Pediatric)

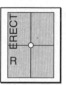

- IR size determined by size of patient, portrait
- Grid >4 inches (10 cm)
- Shortest exposure time possible

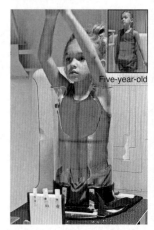

Fig. 9.18 Utilizing Pigg-O-Stat.

Position
- Patient should be erect or seated, legs through openings (when utilizing Pigg-O-Stat).
- Arms should be above head, side body clamps firmly in place (when utilizing Pigg-O-Stat).
- Center IR to CR.

Parental Assistance: Use only if necessary. Have the parent hold arms overhead with one hand, and with other hand hold legs to prevent rotation of pelvis or thorax (provide a lead apron and gloves).

Central Ray
- *Newborn–1 year old:* CR to 1 inch (2.5 cm) above umbilicus
- *Older child:* CR ≈1–2 inches (2.5–5 cm) (depending on the height of the child) above the level of the iliac crest

Minimum SID: 40 inches (100 cm)

Collimation Field Size: Collimate on four sides to area of interest to include soft tissue margins

Respiration: Exposure on expiration, or during least movement

kVp Range:					60–75	
	cm	kVp	mA	Time	mAs	SID	Exposure Indicator
S							
M							
L							

Textbook, 11th ed, p. 653

AP Supine and Erect: Abdomen (Pediatric)

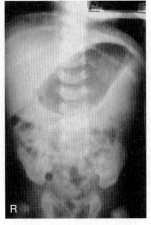

Fig. 9.19 AP supine abdomen.   **Fig. 9.20** Erect AP abdomen.

Evaluation Criteria

Anatomy Demonstrated

- **AP supine and erect:** Entire contents of abdomen are demonstrated including gas patterns, air-fluid levels, and soft tissue if not obscured by excessive fluid in distended abdomen.

Position

- **AP supine and erect:** Diaphragm to symphysis pubis included, if possible; no rotation

Exposure

- Optimal image receptor exposure and contrast allow visualization of soft tissue structures and skeletal structures; no motion

RAO: Esophagogram

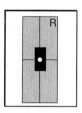

- 14 × 17 inches (35 × 43 cm), portrait
- Grid

Position
- Patient should be recumbent (preferred) or erect.
- Rotate body 35°–40° from prone position onto right side, right arm down, left arm up; hold cup of barium with left hand, straw in mouth.

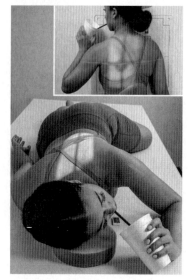

Fig. 9.21 35°–40° RAO for esophagus (barium swallow).

- Center and align thorax to midline of IR or table.
- Top of IR should be ≈2 inches (5 cm) above level of shoulder.

Central Ray: CR ⊥ to center of IR at level of T6 (2 to 3 inches [5 to 8 cm] inferior to jugular notch)

SID: 40 inches (100 cm)

Collimation Field Size: Collimate on four sides to area of (≈ 5–6 inches [12–15 cm] wide) to include soft tissue margins

Respiration: With thin barium, expose while swallowing (after three or four swallows). With thick barium, expose immediately after swallowing. The patient generally does not breathe immediately after a swallow.

	cm	kVp	mA	Time	mAs	SID	Exposure Indicator
kVp Range:			110–125				
S							
M							
L							

Textbook, 11th ed, p. 490

Lateral: Esophagogram

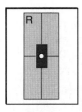

- 14 × 17 inches (35 × 43 cm) portrait
- Grid

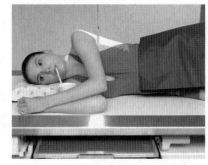

Fig. 9.22 R lateral esophagogram (barium swallow).

Position

- Patient should be recumbent (preferred) or erect.
- Use right lateral position, right arm and shoulder up and forward (holding cup of barium).
- Center and align midcoronal plane to midline of IR or table.
- Top of IR should be ≈2 inches (5 cm) above top of shoulder.

Central Ray: CR ⊥ to center of IR at level of T6 (2 to 3 inches [5 to 8 cm] inferior to jugular notch)

SID: 40 inches (100 cm) or 72 inches (180 cm) if performed erect

Collimation Field Size: Collimate on two sides along lateral borders to area ≈5–6 inches [12–15 cm] wide

Respiration: With thin barium, expose while the patient is swallowing (after three or four swallows). With thick barium, expose immediately after the patient swallows. The patient generally does not breathe immediately after a swallow.

	cm	kVp	mA	Time	mAs	SID	Exposure Indicator
kVp Range:					110–125		
S							
M							
L							

Textbook, 11th ed, p. 491

RAO and Lateral: Esophagogram

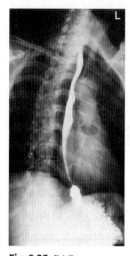

Fig. 9.23 RAO esophagogram.

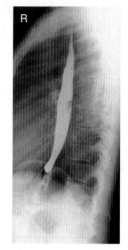

Fig. 9.24 Right lateral esophagogram.

Evaluation Criteria

Anatomy Demonstrated

- **RAO:** Esophagus visible between vertebral column and heart
- **Lateral:** Entire esophagus visible between thoracic spine and heart

Position

- **RAO:** Entire esophagus filled with contrast media and not superimposed over spine
- **Lateral:** No rotation; superimposition of posterior ribs, entire esophagus filled with contrast media

Exposure

- Optimal image receptor exposure and contrast allow visualization of borders of contrast-filled esophagus; no motion.
- Sharp structural margins

AP (PA): Esophagogram

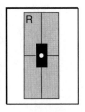

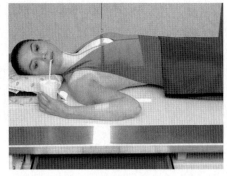

Fig. 9.25 AP esophagogram (barium swallow).

- 14 × 17 inches (35 × 43 cm), portrait
- Grid

Position

- Patient should be erect or supine; supine is preferred (may be performed PA if erect).
- Place patient's arms near the head, with the elbows flexed and superimposed.
- Align **midcoronal plane to midline** of IR or table.
- Place shoulders and hips in a true lateral position.
- Top of IR should be ≈2 inches (5 cm) above top of shoulder.
- Place left arm at side, holding cup of barium with right hand, straw in mouth.

Central Ray: CR ⊥ to center of IR at level of T6 (2 to 3 inches [5 to 8 cm] inferior to jugular notch)

SID: 40 inches (100 cm) or 72 inches (180 cm) if performed erect

Collimation Field Size: Collimate on two sides along lateral borders to area ≈5–6 inches (12–15 cm) wide

Respiration: With thin barium, expose while patient is swallowing (after three or four swallows). With thick barium, expose immediately after patient swallows.

	cm	kVp	mA	Time	mAs	SID	Exposure Indicator
kVp Range:				110–125			
S							
M							
L							

Textbook, 11th ed, p. 492

RAO: Upper GI (Stomach)

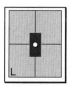

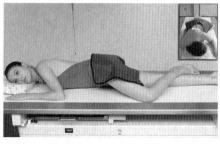

- 10 × 12 inches (24 × 30) portrait
- Grid

Fig. 9.26 40°–70° RAO, upper GI (stomach).

Position

- Patient should be semiprone; rotate 40°–70° from prone with right anterior body against IR or table (more rotation is often required for hypersthenic patients, and less is required for asthenic patients).
- Place right arm down and left **arm flexed** at elbow and up by the patient's head; partially flex left hip and knee.
- Align and center patient to CR.

Central Ray: CR ⊥ to IR

Sthenic: Center to duodenal bulb at level of L1 (≈1–2 inches [2.5–5 cm]) above lower ribs and midway between spine and upside left lateral abdominal border, 45°–55° oblique from prone.

Hypersthenic: Center 2 inches (5 cm) above level of L1 and nearer midline, ≈70° oblique.

Asthenic: Center ≈2 inches (5 cm) below level of L1, ≈40° oblique.

SID: 40 inches (100 cm)

Collimation Field Size: Collimate on four sides to area of interest to include soft tissue margins

Respiration: Exposure at end of expiratio006E

		kVp Range:				110–125

90–100 kVp (Double Contrast)
80–90 kVp (Water-Soluble Contrast Media)

	cm	kVp	mA	Time	mAs	SID	Exposure Indicator
S							
M							
L							

Textbook, 11th ed, p. 494

PA: Upper GI (Stomach)

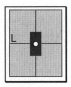

- 14 × 17 inches (35 × 43 cm), or 10 × 12 inches (24 × 30 cm), portrait
- Grid

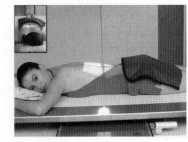

Fig. 9.27 PA upper GI (stomach).

Position
- Patient prone, arms up beside head
- Align MSP to CR and IR

Central Ray: CR ⊥, centered as follows:

Sthenic: Center to pylorus and duodenal bulb at level of L1 (≈1–2 inches [2.5–5 cm]) above lower ribs and ≈1 inch (2.5 cm) to left of vertebral column.

Hypersthenic: Center 2 inches (5 cm) above level of L1 nearer midline.

Asthenic: Center ≈2 inches (5 cm) below level of T1 and nearer midline.

SID: 40 inches (100 cm)

Collimation Field Size: Collimate on four sides to area of interest to include soft tissue margins

Respiration: Exposure at end of expiration

		kVp Range:				110–125

90–100 kVp (Double Contrast)
80–90 kVp (Water-Soluble Contrast Media)

	cm	kVp	mA	Time	mAs	SID	Exposure Indicator
S							
M							
L							

Textbook, 11th ed, p. 495

PA and RAO: Upper GI (Stomach)

Evaluation Criteria

Anatomy Demonstrated

- **PA:** Entire stomach and duodenum
- **RAO:** Entire stomach and C-loop of duodenum

Position

- **PA:** Body and pylorus centered and barium filled
- **RAO:** Pylorus and duodenal bulb in profile and barium filled

Exposure

- Optimal image receptor exposure and contrast allow visualization of gastric folds without overexposing other structures; no motion.
- Sharp structural margins

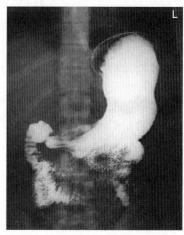

Fig. 9.28 PA.

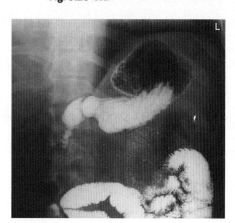

Fig. 9.29 RAO.

Right Lateral: Upper GI (Stomach)

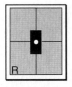

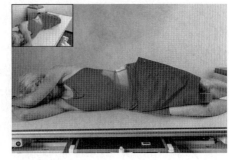

- 10 × 12 inches
  (24 × 30 cm),
  portrait
- Grid

Fig. 9.30 Right lateral upper GI (stomach).

Position

- Patient should be recumbent on right side, arms up, hips and knees partially flexed.
- Align and center patient and IR to CR.

Central Ray: CR ⊥ to the IR

Sthenic: Center to duodenal bulb at level of L1, and 1–1.5 inches (2.5–4 cm) anterior to midcoronal plane (near midway between anterior border of vertebrae and anterior abdomen).

Hypersthenic: Center ≈2 inches (5 cm) above L1.

Asthenic: Center ≈2 inches (5 cm) below L1.

SID: 40 inches (100 cm)

Collimation Field Size: Collimate on four sides to area of interest to include soft tissue margins

Respiration: Exposure at end of expiration

	kVp Range:					110–125
					90–100 kVp (Double Contrast)	
					80–90 kVp (Water-Soluble Contrast Media)	

	cm	kVp	mA	Time	mAs	SID	Exposure Indicator
S							
M							
L							

Textbook, 11th ed, p. 496

Abdomen and Common Contrast Media Procedures

9

AP: Upper GI (Stomach)

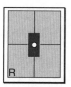

- 14 × 17 inches (35 × 43 cm), portrait
- Grid

Fig. 9.31 AP supine, inset AP Trendelenburg, upper GI (stomach). The Trendelenburg position best demonstrates a hiatal hernia.

Position

- Patient supine or erect, arms at side
- Align and center MSP and IR to CR

Central Ray: CR ⊥ to IR, centered to 1–2 inches (2.5–5 cm) to left of MSP

Sthenic: Center to level of L1 (midway between xiphoid process and level of lower lateral ribs), midway between midline and left lateral margin of abdomen.

Hypersthenic: Center ≈2 inches (5 cm) above level of L1.

Asthenic: Center ≈2 inches (5 cm) below level of L1 and nearer midline.

SID: 40 inches (100 cm)

Collimation Field Size: Collimate on four sides to area of interest to include soft tissue margins

Respiration: Exposure at end of expiration

---

kVp Range:						110–125
					90–100 kVp (Double Contrast)
					80–90 kVp (Water-Soluble Contrast Media)

	cm	kVp	mA	Time	mAs	SID	Exposure Indicator
S							
M							
L							

Textbook, 11th ed, p. 498

Lateral and AP: Upper GI

Evaluation Criteria

Anatomy Demonstrated

- **Right lateral:** Entire stomach, duodenum and retrogastric space demonstrated
- **AP:** Entire stomach and C-loop of duodenum; diaphragm included to r/o hiatal hernia

Position

- **Right lateral:** Pylorus and C-loop of duodenum demonstrated; **no rotation;** evident by aligned vertebral bodies
- **AP:** Fundus centered and barium filled

Exposure

- Optimal image receptor exposure and contrast allow visualization of gastric folds without overexposing other structures; no motion.
- Sharp structural margins

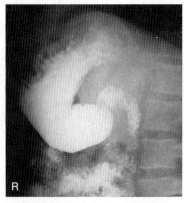

Fig. 9.32 Right lateral upper GI.

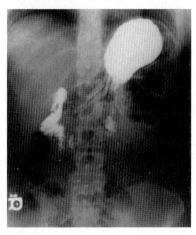

Fig. 9.33 AP upper GI.

LPO: Upper GI (Stomach)

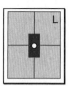

- 10 × 12 inches (24 × 30 cm), portrait
- Grid

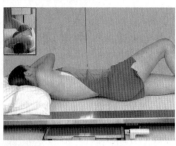

Fig. 9.34 30°–60° LPO, upper GI (stomach).

Position

- Patient should be recumbent with body rotated into an LPO position (0°–60° oblique*) left side down; partially flex right knee.
- Extend left arm from body, and raise right arm high across chest to grasp end of table for support.
- Center patient and IR to CR.

Central Ray: CR ⊥ to IR, centered to left half of abdomen

Sthenic: Center to L1 (midway between xiphoid process and level of lower lateral ribs) and midway between midline of body and left lateral margin of abdomen, 45° oblique.

Hypersthenic: Center ≈2 inches (5 cm) above L1, 60° oblique.

Asthenic: Center ≈2 inches (5 cm) below L1 and nearer midline, 30° oblique.

SID: 40 inches (100 cm)

Collimation Field Size: Collimate on four sides to area of interest to include soft tissue margins

Respiration: Exposure at end of expiration

*Up to 60° for hypersthenic patients and 30° for asthenic patients.

kVp Range:						110–125
						90–100 kVp (Double Contrast)
						80–90 kVp (Water-Soluble Contrast Media)

	cm	kVp	mA	Time	mAs	SID	Exposure Indicator
S							
M							
L							

Textbook, 11th ed, p. 497

LPO: Upper GI (Stomach)

Evaluation Criteria

Anatomy Demonstrated
- Entire stomach and duodenum; unobstructed view of duodenal bulb

Position
- Fundus is barium filled; gas-filled duodenal bulb seen for double-contrast study.
- Duodenal bulb in profile

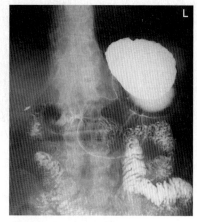

Fig. 9.35 LPO upper GI.

Exposure
- Optimal image receptor exposure and contrast allow visualization of gastric folds without overexposing other structures; no motion.
- Sharp structural and gastric organ margins

AP (PA): Small Bowel

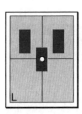

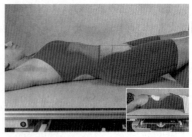

A common routine includes images at 15- or 30-minute intervals until barium reaches ileocecal valve.

Fig. 9.36 AP (PA) small bowel (15 or 30 minutes).

- 14 × 17 inches (35 × 43 cm), portrait
- Grid
- Time indicators visible on image(s)

Position
- Preferably patient should be prone (may be taken AP supine, if necessary).
- MSP should be aligned to midline of table; no rotation.
- Place arms up beside head with legs extended and support provided under the ankles.
- Center patient and IR to iliac crest (center higher on early IRs).

Central Ray: CR ⊥ to IR, to center of IR, ≈2 inches (5 cm) above level of iliac crest for early IRs (15 or 30 minutes), and at iliac crest for later images

SID: 40 inches (100 cm)

Collimation Field Size: Collimate on four sides to area of interest to include soft tissue margins

Respiration: Exposure at end of full expiration

Note: Imaging series and technical factors are similar for enteroclysis and intubation procedures.

	cm	kVp	mA	Time	mAs	SID	Exposure Indicator
S							
M							
L							

kVp Range: 110–125

Textbook, 11th ed, p. 525

PA (AP): Barium Enema

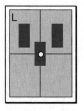

- 14 × 17 inches (35 × 43 cm), portrait
- Grid

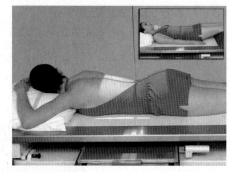

Fig. 9.37 PA barium enema.

Position

- Patient should be prone (PA) or supine (AP).
- Patient should be aligned and centered to midline of table; no rotation.
- Center IR to level of iliac crest (see ***Note***).

Central Ray: CR ⊥ to IR, to center of IR, at level of iliac crest

Note: For long torsed or hypersthenic patients, the use of two IRs may be necessary, placed landscape if the entire large intestine is to be included (one centered for the lower abdomen and one for the upper abdomen).

SID: 40 inches (100 cm)

Collimation Field Size: Collimate on four sides to area of interest to include soft tissue margins

Respiration: Exposure at full expiration

	cm	kVp	mA	Time	mAs	SID	Exposure Indicator
kVp Range:							110–125
						90–100 kVp (Double Contrast)	
						80–90 kVp (Water-Soluble Contrast Media)	
S							
M							
L							

Textbook, 11th ed, p. 527

PA (AP): Barium Enema

Evaluation Criteria

Anatomy Demonstrated

- The transverse colon should be primarily barium filled on the PA and air filled on the AP with a double-contrast study.
- Entire large intestine is demonstrated, including left colic flexure and rectum.

Position

- Transverse colon primarily filled with barium (PA) and gas filled on AP
- **No rotation;** evident by symmetry of ala of ilium and lumbar vertebra

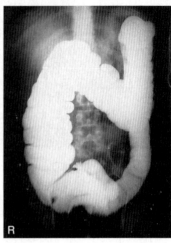

Fig. 9.38 PA single-contrast BE.

Exposure

- Optimal image receptor exposure and contrast allow visualization of mucosa without overexposing other structures; no motion.
- Sharp structural margins

RAO and LAO (RPO and LPO): Barium Enema

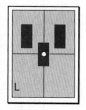

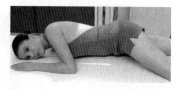

Fig. 9.39 35°–45° RAO barium enema.

Right and left oblique projections are commonly performed.
- 14 × 17 inches (35 × 43 cm), portrait
- Grid

Position
- Patient should be semiprone (PA) or semisupine (AP), rotated 35°–45°; a positioning sponge can be used to help align the upper body into the correct position.
- Align and center abdomen to midline of table.
- IR should be centered to level of iliac crest (include rectal area).

Fig. 9.40 35°–45° LPO.

Central Ray: CR ⊥ to center of IR (at level 1 inch [2.5 cm] above iliac crest) ≈1 inch (2.5 cm) to the left of the MSP

Note: Many patients require a second IR centered ≈2 inches (5 cm) higher if the left colic flexure is to be included—most important on LAO or RPO (determine departmental routine).

SID: 40 inches (100 cm)

Collimation Field Size: Collimate on four sides to area of interest to include soft tissue margins

Respiration: Exposure at expiration

kVp Range:	110–125 kVp (Single Contrast)
	90–100 kVp (Double Contrast)
	80–90 kVp (Water-Soluble Contrast Media)

	cm	kVp	mA	Time	mAs	SID	Exposure Indicator
S							
M							
L							

Textbook, 11th ed, pp. 528–530

RAO and LAO (RPO and LPO): Barium Enema

Evaluation Criteria

Anatomy Demonstrated

- **LPO/RAO:** Right colic flexure and ascending and sigmoid colon
- **RPO/LAO:** Left colic flexure and descending colon

Position

- Spine parallel to the edge of the image
- **LPO/RAO:** Right colic flexure and ascending colon in profile
- **RPO/LAO:** Left colic flexure in profile and descending colon in profile

Exposure

- Optimal image receptor exposure and contrast allows visualization of mucosa without overexposing other structures; no motion.
- Sharp structural margins

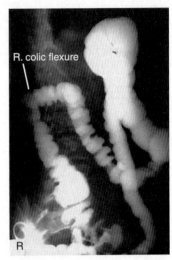

Fig. 9.41 RAO (centered high).

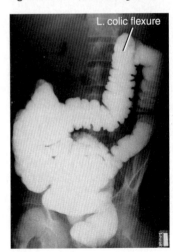

Fig. 9.42 RPO.

Lateral Rectum (Ventral Decubitus): Barium Enema

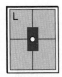

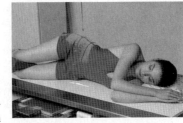

Fig. 9.43 Left lateral for rectum.

Alternative ventral decubitus projection is often performed for double-contrast studies.

- 10 × 12 inches (24 × 30 cm), portrait
- Grid
- Compensating filter for more uniform density on ventral decubitus lateral

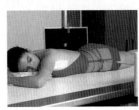

Fig. 9.44 Ventral decubitus lateral rectum (alternate projection with double-contrast examination).

Position

- Patient should be recumbent in true lateral position.
- Center midaxillary plane to midline of table, with knees and hips partially flexed.
- Center patient and IR to CR.

Central Ray: CR ⊥ to IR, to level of ASIS, centered to midcoronal plane (midway between ASIS and posterior sacrum). CR is horizontal for ventral decubitus.

SID: 40 inches (100 cm)

Collimation Field Size: Collimate on four sides to area of interest to include soft tissue margins

Respiration: Exposure at expiration

kVp Range:		110–125 kVp (Single Contrast)	90–100 kVp (Double Contrast)			80–90 kVp (Water-Soluble Contrast Media)	

	cm	kVp	mA	Time	mAs	SID	Exposure Indicator
S							
M							
L							

Textbook, 11th ed, p. 531

Lateral Decubitus (Double Contrast): Barium Enema

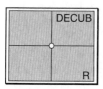

Right and left lateral decubitus are commonly performed as part of a double-contrast series.

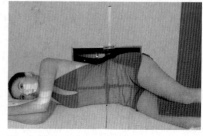

Fig. 9.45 Right lateral decubitus (AP).

- 14 × 17 inches (35 × 43 cm), portrait to patient
- Grid
- Compensating filter placed on upside of abdomen

Position

- Patient should be on side, arms up, knees partially flexed, back against IR or table.
- MSP aligned and centered to centerline of IR (and CR); no rotation (lock wheels if stretcher is used)
- IR centered to level of iliac crest

Central Ray: CR horizontal to center of IR (to level of iliac crest at MSP)

SID: 40 inches (100 cm)

Collimation Field Size: Collimate on four sides to area of interest to include soft tissue margins

Respiration: Exposure at full expiration

kVp Range:			90–100 (Double-Contrast Study)			
	cm	kVp	mA	Time	mAs	SID	Exposure Indicator
S							
M							
L							

Textbook, 11th ed, p. 532

AP (PA) Axial: Barium Enema

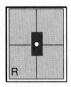

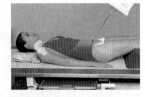

Fig. 9.46 AP axial—CR 30°–45° cephalad.

- 14 × 17 inches (35 × 43 cm), portrait
- Grid

Position

Supine (AP) or Prone (PA): Patient aligned and centered to midline

Alternate Oblique: LPO or RAO: Oblique patient 30°–40°

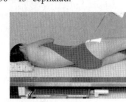

Fig. 9.47 35° LPO axial— CR 30°–40° cephalad.

Central Ray: CR 30°–40° cephalad for AP; 30°–40° caudad for PA

AP Axial: CR to 2 inches (5 cm) inferior to ASIS

PA Axial: CR to enter at level of ASIS

LPO Axial: CR 2 inches (5 cm) inferior and 2 inches (5 cm) medial to right ASIS

SID: 40 inches (100 cm)

Collimation Field Size: Collimate on four sides to area of interest to include soft tissue margins

Respiration: Exposure at full expiration

kVp Range:	110–125 kVp (Single Contrast)
	90–100 kVp (Double Contrast)
	80–90 kVp (Water-Soluble Contrast Media)

	cm	kVp	mA	Time	mAs	SID	Exposure Indicator
S							
M							
L							

Textbook, 11th ed, pp. 535 and 536

Lateral Decubitus and AP (PA) Axial: Barium Enema

Evaluation Criteria

Anatomy Demonstrated

- **Lateral decubitus:** Entire large intestine demonstrated
- **AP/PA axial:** Elongated view of rectosigmoid colon

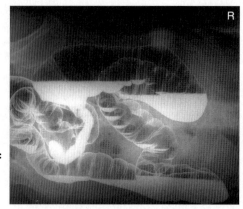

Fig. 9.48 Left lateral decubitus.

Position

- **Lateral decubitus: No rotation** evident by symmetry of pelvis and ribs
- **AP/PA axial:** Less superimposition between rectum and sigmoid colon

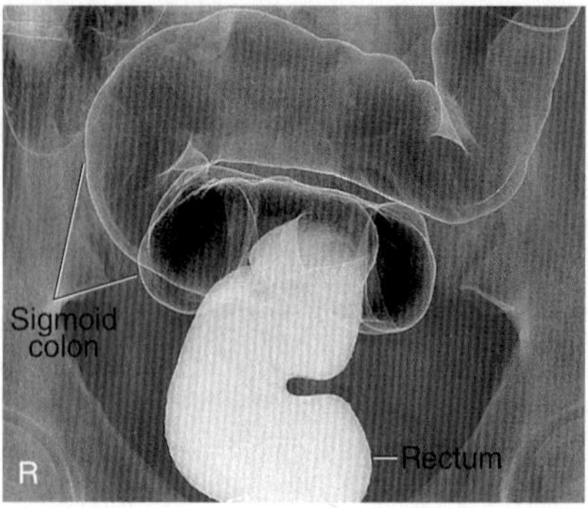

Fig. 9.49 AP axial.

Exposure

- Optimal image receptor exposure and contrast allows visualization of mucosa without overexposing other structures; no motion.
- Sharp structural margins

AP (PA) Scout and Series: Intravenous Urogram (IVU)

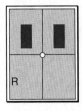

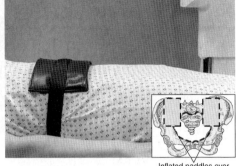

Fig. 9.50 AP IVU with ureteric compression.

Inflated paddles over outer pelvic brim

- 14 × 17 inches (35 × 43 cm), portrait 14 × 17 inches (35 × 43 cm), for nephrotomogram, landscape
- Grid
- Include minute markers, where applicable.
- Note that early images may include nephrotomogram.

Position

- Patient should be supine, MSP aligned and centered to midline of table; support placed under knees; no rotation.
- Include symphysis pubis on bottom of IR without cutting off upper kidneys.

Central Ray

- CR ⊥ to center of IR, at level of iliac crest, or 1–2 inches (2.5–5 cm) above crests on long-torso patients with second smaller IR landscape for bladder area, to include symphysis pubis on lower border of IR
- *Nephrogram:* Center CR midway between xiphoid process and iliac crest.

SID: 40 inches (100 cm)

Collimation Field Size: Collimate on four sides to area of interest to include soft tissue margins

Respiration: Exposure at end of full expiration

	cm	kVp	mA	Time	mAs	SID	Exposure Indicator
S							
M							
L							

kVp Range: 80–85

Textbook, 11th ed, p. 570

RPO and LPO: IVU

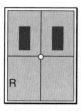

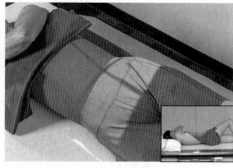

Right and left posterior oblique projections should be part of the routine.

Fig. 9.51 30°—RPO. (*Inset:* LPO.)

- 14 × 17 inches (35 × 43 cm), portrait
- Grid
- Include minute marker(s).

Position
- Patient should be semisupine, 30° oblique to right (or left); flex elevated knee and elbow, as shown, for support (place angled support under back, if needed).
- Align and center abdomen to midline.
- Center IR to level of iliac crest.

Central Ray: CR ⊥ to center of IR, at level of iliac crest
SID: 40 inches (100 cm)
Collimation Field Size: Collimate on four sides to area of interest to include soft tissue margins
Respiration: Exposure at end of full expiration

	cm	kVp	mA	Time	mAs	SID	Exposure Indicator
kVp Range:					80–85		
S							
M							
L							

Textbook, 11th ed, p. 568

AP and RPO: IVU

Evaluation Criteria

Anatomy Demonstrated
- **AP and oblique:** Entire urinary system visualized from renal shadows to symphysis pubis

Position
- **AP:** No rotation; evident by symmetry of iliac wings; symphysis pubis and top of kidneys included
- **Oblique:** Kidney on elevated side in profile; downside ureter away from spine

Exposure
- Optimal image receptor exposure and contrast allow visualization of kidneys and ureters without overexposing other structures; no motion.
- Minute and side markers are visible.

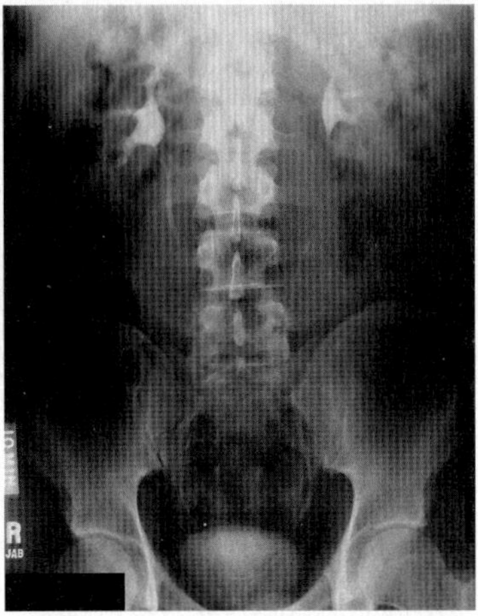

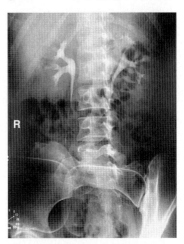

Fig. 9.52 AP—10 minutes (postinjection).

Fig. 9.53 30°—RPO. (From Frank ED, Long BW, Smith BJ: *Merrill's atlas of radiographic positioning and procedures*, ed 12, St. Louis, 2012, Elsevier.)

Abdomen and Common Contrast Media Procedures

9

AP Erect (Postvoid): IVU

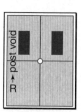

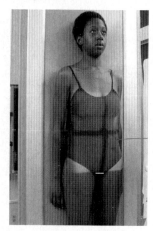

Fig. 9.54 AP erect postvoid.

- 14 × 17 inches (35 × 43 cm), portrait
- Grid
- Erect and postvoid markers

Position

- Patient should be erect, MSP aligned and centered to midline of table, no rotation.
- Center IR to iliac crest—ensure that bladder area, including the symphysis pubis, is included.
- Ensure that the symphysis pubis is included on bottom of the IR.

Central Ray: CR ⊥ to center of IR (at level of iliac crests) or ≈1 inch (2.5 cm) lower than crest to include bladder area

SID: 40 inches (100 cm)

Collimation Field Size: Collimate on four sides to area of interest to include soft tissue margins

Respiration: Exposure at end of full expiration

	cm	kVp	mA	Time	mAs	SID	Exposure Indicator
S							
M							
L							

kVp Range: 80–85

Textbook, 11th ed, p. 569

AP Axial: Cystography

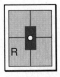

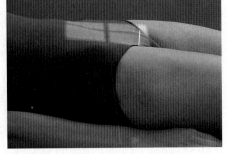

- 14 × 17 inches (35 × 43 cm), portrait for adult
- Grid

Fig. 9.55 AP axial—CR 10°–15° caudad.

Position

- Patient supine, MSP aligned and centered to midline of table, legs fully extended
- Center IR to projected CR

Central Ray: CR 10°–15° caudad, centered to ≈2 inches (5 cm) superior to symphysis pubis at MSP (projects pubis inferiorly to better visualize bladder region)

SID: 40 inches (100 cm)

Collimation Field Size: Collimate on four sides to area of interest to include soft tissue margins

Respiration: Exposure at end of full expiration

	cm	kVp	mA	Time	mAs	SID	Exposure Indicator
kVp Range:					80–90		
S							
M							
L							

Textbook, 11th ed, p. 571

Posterior Oblique (RPO, LPO) and Optional Lateral: Cystography

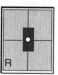

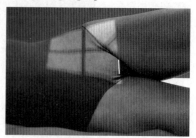

Fig. 9.56 45° RPO.

Note: The cystogram routine may not include a lateral due to the high gonadal dose.
- 14 × 17 inches (35 × 43 cm), portrait
- Grid

Position
- Patient should be semisupine, 45°–60° oblique (60° oblique best demonstrates posterolateral bladder and UV junction).
- Flex elevated arm and leg to support this position.
- Center patient and IR to CR.

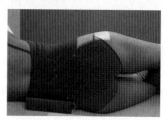

Fig. 9.57 Optional lateral. —CR ⊥, 2 inches (5 cm) superior and post to symphysis pubis.

Central Ray: CR ⊥ to IR, to ≈2 inches (5 cm) superior to symphysis pubis, and 2 inches (5 cm) medial to elevated ASIS, with **10° to 15° caudad** CR angle (to project symphysis pubis inferior to bladder)

SID: 40 inches (100 cm)

Collimation Field Size: Collimate on four sides to area of interest to include soft tissue margins

Respiration: Exposure at expiration

	cm	kVp	mA	Time	mAs	SID	Exposure Indicator
S							
M							
L							

kVp Range: 80–90

Textbook, 11th ed, p. 571

AP and Posterior Oblique: Cystography

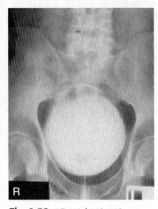

Fig. 9.58 AP axial 10°–15° caudad.

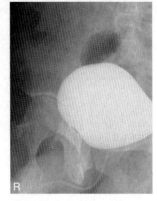

Fig. 9.59 45° posterior oblique.

Evaluation Criteria

Anatomy Demonstrated

- **AP axial and oblique:** Distal ureters, bladder, and proximal urethra

Position

- **AP axial:** Urinary bladder not superimposed by pubic bones
- **Oblique:** Urinary bladder not superimposed by partially flexed leg

Exposure

- Optimal image receptor exposure and contrast allows visualization of urinary bladder without overexposing other structures; no motion.

Abdomen and Common Contrast Media Procedures

9

Mobile (Portables) and Surgical Procedures

Essential Principles for Trauma and Mobile Radiography

The following three principles must be observed for trauma and mobile procedures:

- **Two projections 90° to each other (minimum):** Trauma radiography generally requires two projections taken at 90° (or right angles to each other) while true CR-part-IR alignment is maintained.
- **Entire anatomic structure (or trauma area) on IR:** Trauma radiography mandates that the entire structure being examined should be included on the image to ensure that no pathologic condition is missed. Additional projections must be performed if the entire structure is not seen on the initial image.
- **Maintain the safety of the patient, health care workers, and the public:** Technologists must maintain the safety and well-being of patients, family/friends, and other health care workers during a trauma or mobile radiographic procedure. Safe handling of patients and radiation protection of the patient and others in the immediate vicinity of the exposure is the responsibility of the technologist.
- **Grid Use:** The body part and the central ray (CR) should be centered to the IR to avoid image distortion and grid cut-off. Anatomy thickness and kVp range are deciding factors for whether a grid is to be used. Virtual grid technology may eliminate the need for a physical grid.

AP Chest (Supine and Semierect): Mobile

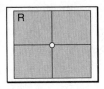

Warning: With possible spinal injury or severe trauma, do not attempt to move the patient.

- Collimation Field Size: 14 × 17 inches (35 × 43 cm), landscape or portrait
- Grid > 4 cm (10 cm)

Position

- Cover IR with plastic case, and center to patient with top of IR approximately 2 inches (5 cm) above shoulders.

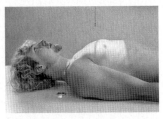

Fig. 10.1 Supine AP chest.

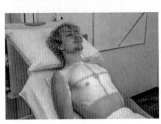

Fig. 10.2 Semierect AP chest.

- Patient should be supine; elevate head of bed, if possible, into seated or semierect position.
- Ensure no rotation of patient.
- If patient condition allows, rotate shoulders forward to move scapulae out of lung fields.

Central Ray

- Direct CR 3–4 inches (8–10 cm) below jugular notch at level of T7
- CR 3°–5° caudal from ⊥ to IR so as to be ⊥ to sternum (prevents clavicles from obscuring apices of lungs)
- If patient is able to attain only a semierect position, the CR must be angled to maintain the ⊥ relationship with the IR.

SID: 48–72 inches (120–180 cm); use greater SID, if possible

Respiration: Expose after second full inspiration.

	cm	kVp	mA	Time	mAs	SID	Exposure Indicator
						90–125*	
S							
M							
L							

kVp Range: 90–125*

Textbook, 11th ed, p. 585

*Lower kVp for nongrid procedures

AP Supine Abdomen (KUB): Mobile

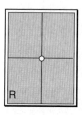

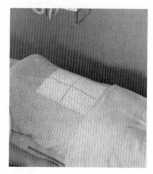

Warning: With possible spinal injury or severe trauma, do not attempt to move the patient.

- Collimation Field Size: 14 × 17 inches (35 × 43 cm), portrait
- Grid

Fig. 10.3 AP supine abdomen.

Position

- Cover IR with plastic case.
- Center IR to patient at level of iliac crest.
- Place supports under IR, if needed, to ensure IR is level and ⊥ to CR (prevents patient rotation and grid cutoff).

Central Ray: CR ⊥ to IR, centered to IR at level of iliac crest

SID: 40 inches (100 cm)

Respiration: Expose on expiration.

	cm	kVp	mA	Time	mAs	SID	Exposure Indicator
S							
M							
L							

kVp Range: 70–90*

Textbook, 11th ed, p. 587

Lateral Decubitus (Abdomen): Mobile

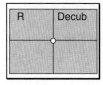

Left lateral best demonstrates free air in right upper abdomen. Must include diaphragm.

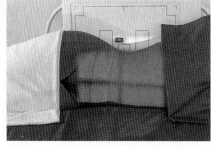

Fig. 10.4 AP left lateral decubitus abdomen.

- Collimation Field Size: 14 × 17 inches (35 × 43 cm), landscape (to anatomy)
- Grid
- Decubitus and side marker

Position

- Patient should be on the left (or right if indicated) side with support, as shown, to prevent sinking into soft bed.
- Center of IR 2 inches (5 cm) above level of iliac crest to include diaphragm.
- Ensure no rotation and that the IR plane is ⊥ to CR.

Central Ray: Horizontal CR to center of IR 2 inches (5 cm) above iliac crest

SID: 40 inches (100 cm)

Respiration: Expose on expiration.

Note: Have patient on side 5 minutes (minimum) before exposure; a period of 10–20 minutes is preferred. Ensure that the diaphragm and "up" side of abdomen are included.

kVp Range:					70–90		
	cm	kVp	mA	Time	mAs	SID	Exposure Indicator
S							
M							
L							

Textbook, 11th ed, p. 587

Mobile (Portables) and Surgical Procedures

10

327

AP Pelvis or Hip: Mobile

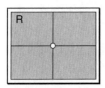

Warning: Do not attempt to rotate leg internally if hip fracture is suspected.

Collimation Field Size
- **Pelvis**: 14 × 17 inches (35 × 43 cm), landscape
- **Hip only**: 10 × 12 inches (24 × 30 cm), portrait
- Grid

Position: Pelvis
- Cover IR with plastic case, slide IR under patient, centered landscape to patient
- Top of IR ≈1 inch (2.5 cm) above iliac crest
- Ensure no rotation of patient (equal ASIS distances to IR).
- Internally rotate both legs 15° (see Warning above).

Central Ray: CR ⊥ midway between ASIS and symphysis pubis

AP Hip:

Warning: Do not attempt to rotate leg internally if hip fracture is suspected.

Center CR and IR to hip region (2 inches [5 cm] medial to ASIS at level of greater trochanter)

SID: 40 inches (100 cm)
Respiration: Suspend during exposure.

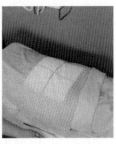

Fig. 10.5 AP pelvis (trauma hip without leg rotation).

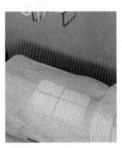

Fig. 10.6 AP hip (with leg rotation).

	cm	kVp	mA	Time	mAs	SID	Exposure Indicator
kVp Range:	Distal Femur	75–90 kVp					
	Proximal Femur/Pelvis	75–90 kVp					
S							
M							
L							

Textbook, 11th ed, pp. 597 and 598

Textbook, 11th ed, pp. 597 and 598

328

Mobile (Portables) and Surgical Procedures

10

Axiolateral Hip (Danelius-Miller Method): Mobile

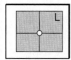

- Collimation Field Size: 10 × 12 inches (24 × 30 cm), landscape (long axis of IR aligned to long axis of femur)
- Grid

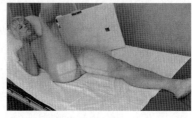

Fig. 10.7 Axiolateral hip.

Position

- Patient should be supine.
- Place folded towels or support under the affected hip.
- Place vertical grid against patient's side with top of IR at the level of the iliac crest with face of grid parallel to femoral neck and ⊥ to CR.
- Elevate opposite leg. (**DO NOT** support leg/foot on collimator or tube because of risk for burns or electrical shock.)
- Internally rotate affected leg (see Warning above).

Central Ray: Horizontal CR angled to be ⊥ to IR and femoral neck

SID: 40 inches (100 cm)

Respiration: Suspend during exposure.

	cm	kVp	mA	Time	mAs	SID	Exposure Indicator
kVp Range:				75–90			
S							
M							
L							

Textbook, 11th ed, p. 598

Modified Axiolateral Hip and Proximal Femur
(Clements-Nakayama Method): Mobile

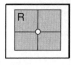

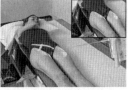

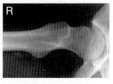

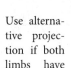

Use alternative projection if both limbs have **Fig. 10.8** Modified axiolateral projection. **Fig. 10.9** Lateral proximal femur (modified axiolateral projection).

limited movement and the inferosuperior projection cannot be obtained.

- 10 × 12 inches (24 × 30 cm), landscape
- Grid (aligned to CR angle to prevent grid cutoff)

Position

- Patient should be supine, affected side near edge of table with both legs fully extended.
- Provide pillow for head, and place arms across superior chest.
- Maintain leg in neutral (anatomical) position.
- Rest IR on extended bucky tray, which places the bottom edge of the IR about 2 inches (5 cm) below the level of the tabletop.
- Tilt IR approximately 15° from vertical, and adjust alignment of IR to ensure that face of IR is ⊥ to CR to prevent grid cutoff.
- Center centerline of IR to projected CR.

Central Ray: Angle CR **mediolaterally** as needed so that it is ⊥ to and **centered to femoral neck** (≈15°–20° posteriorly from horizontal).

SID: 40 inches (100 cm)

	cm	kVp	mA	Time	mAs	SID	Exposure Indicator
kVp Range:					80–90		
S							
M							
L							

Textbook, 11th ed, p. 295

PA Abdomen (Cholangiogram): Surgical C-Arm

Position and CR

- PA projection (patient supine): Image intensifier should be on top, with the tube below.
- Provide lead aprons or portable shields for all personnel in room.

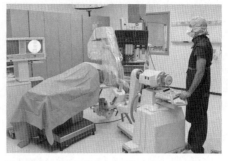

Fig. 10.10 C-arm being positioned for PA hip or abdomen.

- Maintain sterile field.
- Use automatic or manual exposure control.
- Foot pedal allows hands-free operation by physician of fluoroscopic image as displayed on monitor.

Lateral Hip: Surgical C-Arm

Position and CR

- Superoinferior projection
- Horizontal CR, x-ray tube superior, intensifier inferior
- Ensure sterile field.
- Provide lead aprons or shields.
- Background exposure field greatest at tube end; operator should stand back away from tube region.

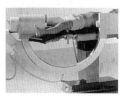

Fig. 10.11 C-arm for lateral hip. (Courtesy Philips Medical System.)

Note: Recommended setup is a reversal of this as an inferosuperior projection because of increased radiation at tube end.

Procedure Notes

Appendix A: Reducing Patient Dose

Six common practices can be used to reduce patient dose during radiographic procedures:

1. **Minimize repeat images:** A primary cause of repeated images is poor communication between the technologist and the patient. The technologist must clearly explain the procedure. Carelessness in positioning and selection of erroneous technique factors are common causes of repeats. Review technical and positioning errors with other technologists and determine corrections before repeating the exposures.

2. **Use correct filtration:** Filtration of the primary x-ray beam reduces exposure to the patient by preferentially absorbing low-energy "unusable" x-rays, which mainly expose the patient's skin and superficial tissue without contributing to image formation.

3. **Use accurate collimation:** The practice of close collimation, to only the area of interest, reduces patient dose by reducing the volume of tissue directly irradiated, and the amount of accompanying scattered radiation is decreased. The technologist must not rely on positive beam limitation (PBL) collimators. PBL will collimate to the size of the image receptor only. Additional collimation is needed to further reduce exposure to surrounding tissues not required for the study.

4. **Shielding:** Radiologic technologists should follow local regulations, department policy and protocol in the use of shielding.

5. **Protect the fetus:** All females of childbearing age should be screened for the possibility of pregnancy before an x-ray examination. The technologist should follow departmental policy and protocol related to imaging pregnant patients.

6. **Select projections and exposure factors appropriate for the examination:** Perform projections (pending department approval) that minimize dose to radiosensitive tissues, such as the breast and eye. A PA projection will greatly reduce dose to these tissues compared with an AP projection. Select exposure factors that use highest allowable kVp and lowest mAs to further reduce patient dose.

Ethical Practice in Digital Imaging: The wide dynamic range of digital imaging enables an acceptable image to be obtained with a broad range of exposure factors. During the evaluation of the quality of an image, the technologist must ensure the exposure indicator is within the recommended range. But do not merely rely on exposure indicator values for the determination of image quality. Use exposure factors that will reduce patient dose while maintaining image quality. Any attempt to process an image with a different algorithm to correct overexposure is not acceptable; it is vital that patient dose be minimized at the outset and that the ALARA (As Low As Reasonably Achievable) principle be upheld.

To maintain dose at a reasonable, consistent level, the following practices are recommended:

- Use protocol-specific kVp ranges and mAs values for all procedures. Use as high an kVp as possible.
- Monitor dose by reviewing all images.
- If the exposure indicator for a given procedure is outside of the acceptable range, review all factors, including kVp, mAs, positioning, collimation, and anatomy. If exposure indicator values are consistently outside of the acceptable range, consult with a supervisor or radiation safety officer (RSO).
- Do not use postprocessing masking in place of preexposure collimation. Collimation improves image quality and reduces patient dose.

Appendix B: Grid Ratio Conversion Chart

New Grid Ratio	Recommended kVp Range	Original Grid Ratio (Original Exposure Factors)				
		Nongrid	5:1 or 6:1	8:1	12:1	16:1
Nongrid	<60–70	1	0.33	0.25	0.20 (0.17)	0.17 (0.14)
5:1 or 6:1	60–75	3	1.00	0.75	0.60	0.50
8:1	70–90	4	1.33	1.00	0.80	0.67
12:1	70–125 (95–125)	5 (6)	1.67	1.25	1.00	0.83
16:1	70–125 (95–125)	6 (7)	2.00	1.50	1.20	1.00

This conversion chart can be used for general grid conversions based on recommended mid-kVp ranges of each grid type. To use this chart, determine the correct conversion factor (multiplication number) by looking down the chart to the new grid being used, and multiply by this factor.

Example: If 7 **mAs** @ 70 kVp is the technique for a shoulder using a 12:1 grid, what mAs should be used with a 5:1 portable grid?

Answer: The conversion factor for converting from 12:1 to 5:1 is **0.6**.

7 mAs × 0.6 = 4.2 mAs @ 70 kVp

To check your answer, convert the other way from a 5:1 to a 12:1 grid. An increase in technique would be needed, and the conversion factor is **1.67** (4.2 mAs × 1.67 = **7 mAs**, the original technique for the 12:1 grid).

Appendix C: Initials (Abbreviations), Technical Terms, and Acronyms

The following are the more common initials (abbreviations) and acronyms used in imaging departments today and used in this pocket handbook and in the 11th edition of the Lampignano/Kendrick textbook.

General Positioning/Anatomy Terms

AC joints	Acromioclavicular joints
AP, PA	Anteroposterior, posteroanterior projections
ASIS	Anterior superior iliac spine (pelvis landmark)
DP, PD	Dorsoplantar and plantodorsal
LAO, RAO	Left and right anterior oblique projections
LPO, RPO	Left and right posterior oblique projections
MCP	Midcoronal plane (plane dividing the body into anterior and posterior halves)
MSP	Midsagittal plane (plane dividing the body into equal right and left halves)
SC joints	Sternoclavicular joints
SI joints	Sacroiliac joints
SMV, VSM	Submentovertex or verticosubmental projections

Abdominal Procedure Terms

BE	Barium enema
CNS	Central nervous system
CSF	Cerebrospinal fluid
CTC	Computed tomography colonoscopy
ERCP	Endoscopic retrograde cholangiopancreatography
GB	Gallbladder
GI, UGI, LGI	Gastrointestinal, upper and lower GI
IVP	Intravenous pyelogram (older term)
IVU	Intravenous urogram (accurate term)
KUB	Kidneys, ureters, bladder (abdomen projection)
NPO	Nil per os (nothing by mouth)
PTC	Percutaneous transhepatic cholangiography
RLQ, LLQ	Right and left lower quadrant
RUQ, LUQ	Right and left upper quadrant
SBS	Small bowel series
VC	Virtual colonoscopy

Technical Terms

AEC	Automatic exposure controls
Analog	Film-screen imaging system
CR	Central ray (for positioning centering)
CR	Computed radiography—using image plates (IP)
CT	Computed tomography
DF	Digital fluoroscopy
DR	Digital radiography (cassetteless)
FS	Focal spot (large or small)
HIS	Hospital information system
IP	Image plates (used with CR)
IR	Image receptor
Landscape	Crosswise (IR orientation to patient)
MRI	Magnetic resonance imaging
OID	Object image receptor distance
PACS	Picture archiving and communications system
PBL	Positive beam limitation (automated collimation)
PET	Positron emission tomography
PSP	Photostimulable phosphor plate receptor (either cassette or cassetteless)
Portrait	Lengthwise (IR orientation to patient)
RIS	Radiology information system
SID	Source image-receptor distance
TT	Tabletop (nonbucky)

Terms Related to Joints of Limbs (Extremities)

ACL, PCL	Anterior and posterior cruciate ligaments (knee)
CMC	Carpometacarpal (wrist)
DIP	Distal interphalangeal (hand or foot)
IP	Interphalangeal (hand or foot)
LCL, MCL	Lateral and medial collateral ligaments (knee)
MCP	Metacarpophalangeal (hand)
MTP	Metatarsophalangeal (foot)
PIP	Proximal interphalangeal (hand or foot)
TMT	Tarsometatarsal (foot)

Terms Related to Cranium and Facial Bones

AML	Acanthiomeatal line
EAM	External acoustic meatus
GAL	Glabelloalveolar line
GML	Glabellomeatal line
IOML	Infraorbital-meatal line
IPL	Interpupillary line
LML	Lips-meatal line
MML	Mentomeatal line
OML	Orbitomeatal line
SOG	Supraorbital groove
TEA	Top of ear attachment
TMJ	Temporomandibular joints